MEDITATION FOR WEIGHT LOSS

How Powerful Meditation, Affirmations, And Healthy Eating Habits Lead To Fat Burn. Stop Emotional Eating For A Natural And Rapid Weight Loss.

American Hypnosis Academy

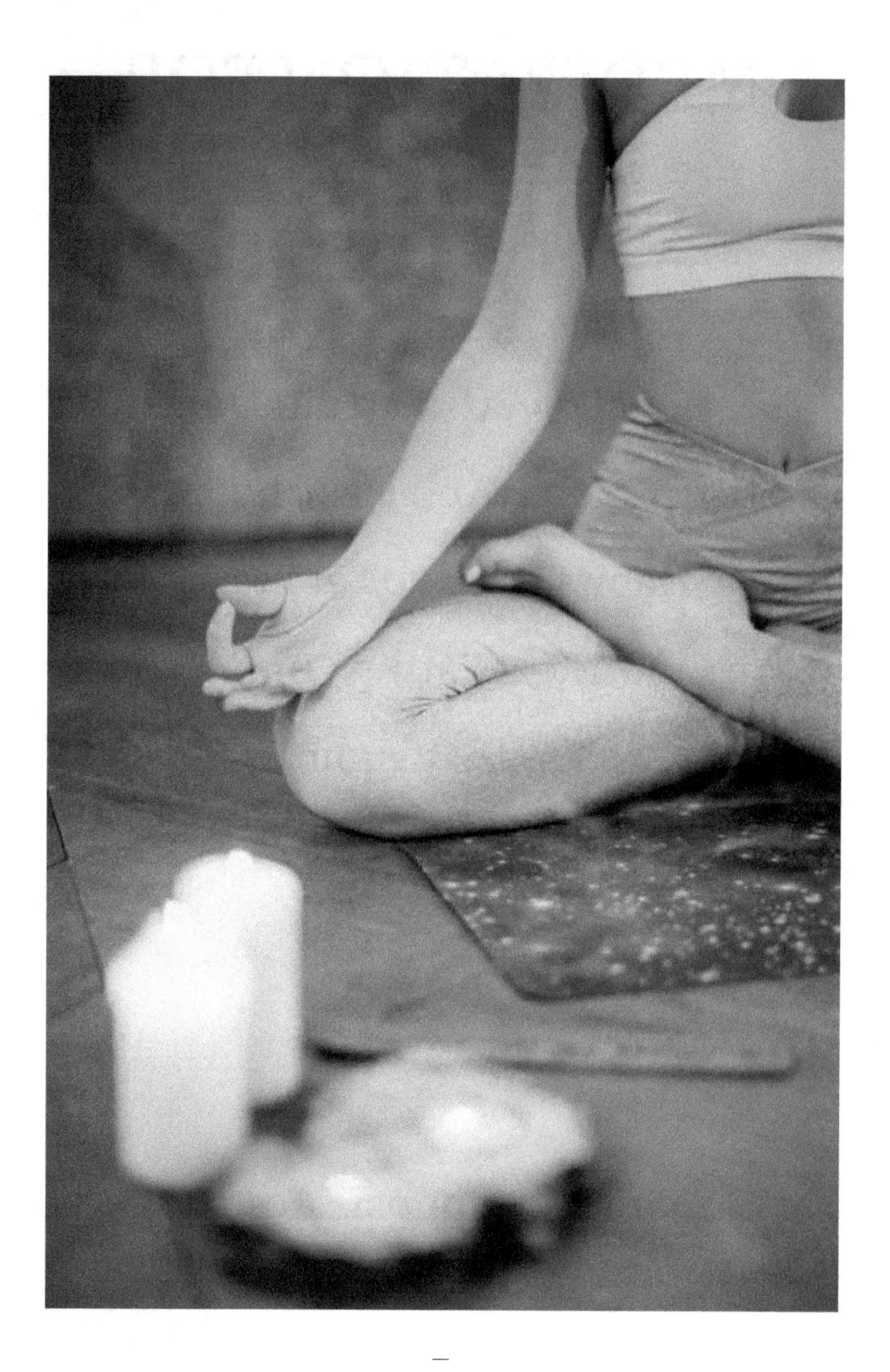

Table of Content

INTRODUCTION 8

MEDITATION: THE BASICS 12
    WHAT IS MEDITATION? 12
    THE EFFECT OF MEDITATION 13
    MEDITATION'S BENEFICIAL MAGIC 16
    THE POWER OF AFFIRMATION 17

WHY MEDITATE? 20
    WHAT ARE THE BENEFITS OF MEDITATION? 20
        It is Good for Our Bodies 20
        Because It's Good for Our Relationships 21
        Because it can Change Our Lives 22
    MYTHS BEHIND MEDITATION 22

WHAT IS BEING MINDFUL? 30
    BENEFITS OF MINDFULNESS FOR YOUR BODY 31

STARTING YOUR MEDITATION JOURNEY 39
    MEDITATION TECHNIQUES YOU CAN USE 39
        Mantra Meditation 39
        Body Scan Meditation 41
        Chakra Meditation 42

WEIGHT LOSS, MEDITATION AND MINDSET: HOW THEY'RE LINKED TO EACH OTHER 45
    THE POWER OF REPEATED WORDS AND THOUGHTS 48

MEDITATION METHODS TO LOSE WEIGHT 52

SIMPLY HEALTHY EATING HABITS 59
    FOODS AND DRINKS 59
        Avoiding processed foods 59
        Avoiding carbs 60
        Eat only the recommended portion of food 61
        Eat lightly cooked food 62

Reduce your sugar intake *63*
Avoid overeating *64*
Drink water regularly *65*

FITNESS STRATEGIES 68

POSITIVE AFFIRMATIONS TO CUT CALORIES 77
AFFIRMATIONS TO CUT CALORIES NATURALLY 77

GUIDED MEDITATION FOR WEIGHT LOSS 84
A SIMPLE DAILY WEIGHT LOSS MEDITATION 85
THE MEDITATION 86

POSITIVE THINKING MEDITATION 90

FAT BURNING MEDITATION 97

MEDITATION AND RELAXATION FOR WEIGHT LOSS 101
MEDITATING SITTING DOWN 102
MEDITATING WHILE STANDING 104
MEDITATING WHILE WALKING 107

CONCLUSION 110

© Copyright 2021 by American Hypnosis Academy - All rights reserved.

The following Book is reproduced below with the goal of providing information that is as accurate and reliable as possible. Regardless, purchasing this Book can be seen as consent to the fact that both the publisher and the author of this book are in no way experts on the topics discussed within and that any recommendations or suggestions that are made herein are for entertainment purposes only. Professionals should be consulted as needed prior to undertaking any of the action endorsed herein.

This declaration is deemed fair and valid by both the American Bar Association and the Committee of Publishers Association and is legally binding throughout the United States.

Furthermore, the transmission, duplication, or reproduction of any of the following work including specific information will be considered an illegal act irrespective of if it is done electronically or in print. This extends to creating a secondary or tertiary copy of the work or a recorded copy and is only allowed with the express written consent from the Publisher. All additional right reserved.

The information in the following pages is broadly considered a truthful and accurate account of facts and as such, any inattention, use, or misuse of the information in question by the reader will render any resulting actions solely under their purview. There are no scenarios in which the publisher or the original author of this work can be in any fashion deemed liable for any hardship or damages that may befall them after undertaking information described herein.

Additionally, the information in the following pages is intended only for informational purposes and should thus be thought of as universal. As befitting its nature, it is presented without assurance regarding its prolonged validity or interim quality. Trademarks that are mentioned are done without written consent and can in no way be considered an endorsement from the trademark holder.

Introduction

Do you battle to get more fit? Have you generally pictured yourself as dainty, alluring, and liberated from any wellbeing conditions welcomed on by abundance weight? Do you want to get certain things throughout your life, just to feel kept down by the body that you have?

Now and again, we battle to get more fit since we don't have the correct mentality to do as such. We expect doing physical things like eating well and practicing being everything necessary. An enormous piece of weight reduction is mental. This may be the most significant piece of all. If you don't have a solid outlook and one that is centered around showing signs of improvement, at that point you may battle to lose the weight. This, yet you may find that you battle since you can't keep the weight off, significantly after you lose it at first.

Weight reduction can be a difficult and overpowering excursion. Many weight reduction assets center generally around your eating routine, which is positively significant however can likewise be overpowering. At the point when you set out on the excursion of weight reduction, you may wind up battling to step away from old propensities that lead to your weight gain in any case. You may end up continually ricocheting to and fro between being "on the cart" and "off the cart," which may prompt you feeling remorseful and battling much more to satisfy your wants of weight reduction.

A weight-loss diet, by definition, requires a reduction in food intake below what the body needs to maintain its current form. There is no real food shortage, but all the built-in mechanisms that ensure our survival record fat loss. This reduction triggers a neural circuit that uses an army of hormones that cause the order of overeating. This mechanism is simply called the famine brain.

Overeating works as the brain's primary reward system for dieting. Unfortunately, researchers have found that weight loss of all kinds uses our neurochemical weapons. If you have too much fat, your body won't know. It only "knows" if you risk losing fat. In a brave attempt to regain homeostasis, our system lowers the hormone levels that signal satiety (leptin and insulin) and pumps the fasting hormone 'ghrelin' into the bloodstream. This hormone results in heightened craving for food leading to extra calorie intake and eventually more weight gain.

Scientists are not yet aware of how the brain and physical starvation system interact to support or override each other. What we know is that many regular diets lead to a mind obsessed with food. Therefore, the root of the problem lies in the brain where this cycle continues.

In this guidebook, we will study self-hypnosis, guided meditation for weight loss, sleep learning system, and different affirmations that can help in reducing weight.

It also covers seemingly ordinary but very influential tricks to get rid of excess fat. We will also learn a few practical habits employing the techniques mentioned above. We will investigate the location of the problem and how it affects us so that we can suggest targeted actions.

Shedding pounds can frequently appear to be overwhelming, particularly in the event that you've stood by too long even to consider beginning the excursion. You won't get results for the time being, and that can be disappointing for a few. Be that as it may, with the utilization of spellbinding, you will have the option to see an adjustment in your negative propensities and self-hurting nourishing way. This contemplation and entrancing will control you through the procedure of tolerance and thankfulness on your excursion to more beneficial and more joyful way of life.

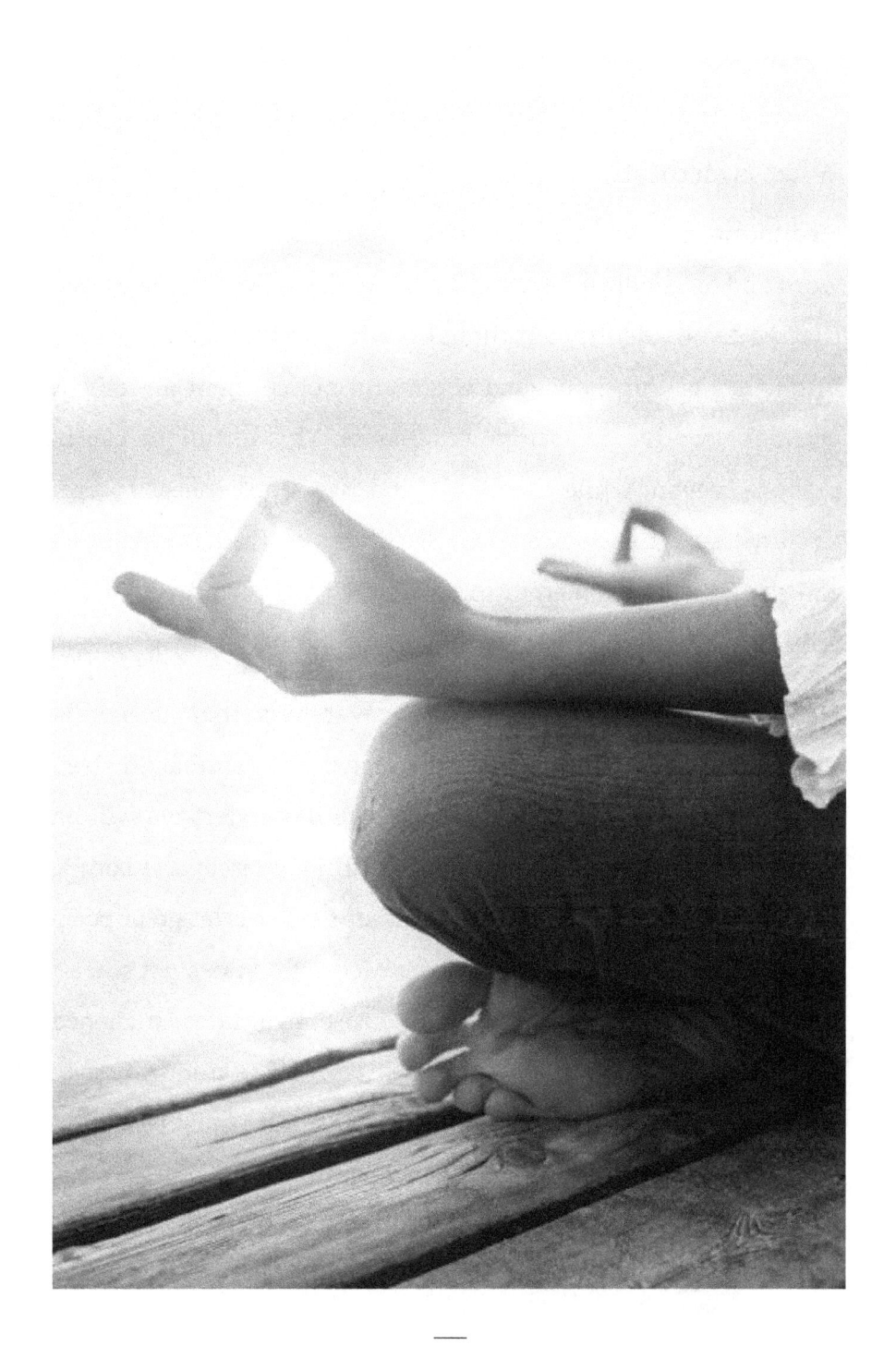

Meditation: The Basics

What is Meditation?

Meditation comes from the word "medicine", which is a Latin word and originally means natural medicine. Meditation signifies that we do not identify our thoughts with the voice and emotions in our heads, but go beyond them and notice them objectively without negative or positive judgments. This technique can be practiced even while cleaning, and we don't need specific circumstances to meditate. If we do something from the heart, we can say that we are meditating. Meditation is the art of entirely redirecting focus to only one thing.

Meditation is a changed state of awareness that cannot be produced by will or forced. In this regard, it is similar to sleep, because the more we want to sleep, the more alert we will be. Meditation usually refers to a state of mind whereby the body is consciously carefree and relaxed, and our spirit is let go of peace and concentration within ourselves. Meditation does not merely imply sitting or lying down for five to ten minutes in silence. Meditation indeed demands mindful work. The mind must be relaxed and balanced. At the same time, the brain must be alert so that it does not allow any disturbing thoughts or desires to penetrate. We begin meditation with our effort. Still, when we delve intensely into ourselves, we see that it is not our individual self that allows us to enter the state of meditation. The Supreme or Creator meditates within and through us, with our deliberate attention and permission.

The aim is to seek peace and freedom from disturbing thoughts. In such cases, the meditator achieves an escape from the environment so that from a psychological point of view, the experience could even be called a changed state of consciousness. When we can make our minds calm and still, we will touch a new existence awakened within us. If our mind is discharged and tranquil, and our entire being becomes an empty vessel, then our internal presence can call upon eternal peace, light, and mercy to flow into and fill this vessel. This happens during meditation.

The Effect of Meditation

Meditation has been used in many cultures for thousands of years because of its numerous benefits: it reduces anxiety, and makes people feel happy. In the short term, meditation has mainly psychological advantages, but in the long run, it has physical outcomes. Those who try meditation can enjoy its benefits in the short term such as balance, greater peace and vitality, and a decreased need for sleep. Physical effects can be experienced in just a few months: among other things, blood pressure may return to normal, or digestion may improve. So, you can imagine how beneficial it can be in the long run.

The University of California's Neuroscience Laboratory has been researching the impacts of meditation on the brain's structure for years. Their most recent research has studied long-term effects in the minds of habitual meditators compared to non-meditators. According to their results, the cerebral cortex of long-term meditators is more marked than that of non-meditators, indicating increased cognitive performance. The Frontiers in Human Neuroscience published research which became a milestone in science because it has long been believed that the brain mass reaches its peak in the early twenties, and then begins to narrow slowly (Bae, Hurl, Hwang, Jung, Kang, Kim, Kwan, Kwon, Lee, Lim, Cho, & Park, 2019). it was a widespread opinion that there was no way to interrupt this process. However, it is now known that the brain retains its plasticity to some extent, and it can physically change as a result of meditation. Earlier studies have shown that for long-time meditators, both gray matter and white matter in the brain have increased in weight. (The former contains the cells of the brain nerve cells; the latter contains the neuronal cell-forming projections). The number of neurons in the cortex changes only very rarely in adulthood. One group of the current research involved 28 men and 22 women, their average age was 51, and they had all been meditating for an average of 20 years. The oldest participant was 71, and the most experienced meditator had been practicing daily for 46 years. The researchers performed MRI scans of participants' brains and compared them to 50 non-meditating members of the control group.

Regular practice can increase the advantages of meditation. According to research, the more practitioners repeated deep breathing techniques and other meditation methods, the more they relieved the symptoms of arthritis, reduced their pain, increased their immune systems, manifested healthier hormone levels, and lowered blood pressure. According to the researchers, this explains that a person's mental state can change his physical condition and gives an added motivation to why traditional Tibetan, Indian, and Ayurveda medicine view meditation and the repetition of mantras as therapeutic.

Hundreds of scientific documents confirm the positive healing and health benefits of meditation. Here are some of them.

During the first twenty minutes of meditation, metabolism is reduced by sixteen percent. The body deeply calms down during transcendental meditation, which is the result of decreased cellular oxygen utilization due to reduced metabolism. It also decreases heart rate and stabilizes blood circulation (Dill beck, & Oren-Johnson, 1987). Besides, the blood pressure decreases, and muscular tension and anxiety consequently disappear. Meditation has proven to be effective in overcoming chronic anxiety and in increasing self-esteem (Apply, Abrams, & Shear, 1989). Meditation is also an effective way to create relaxation and reduce physiological stimulation. The essence of the phenomenon is a decrease in respiratory rate, oxygen consumption and carbon dioxide exhalation. Breathing is not only rarer but more profound, vital capacity increases from resting 450-550 ml to 800-1300 ml (up to 2000 ml for some master meditators) and remains consistent throughout. However, a lower respiratory rate is not offset by deeper breathing, resulting in a 20% reduction in respiratory volume under rest.

Meditation's Beneficial Magic

Meditation has impressive power because we associate emotions coming from the depths of the soul with conscious thought. In meditation, the individual is brought into the same frequency as the origin of the Inner Self, that is, the Universe itself, and thus is directly connected to the consciousness sphere of the Universe. In this state, there is no time limit, so the visualized fulfillment can immediately expand to the physical level. As a result of regular meditation, we obtain numerous benefits in a physical and mental sense. We will be healthier because when we focus on our breathing, our blood pressure drops, our heart rate slows down; consequently, we become calmer. It helps us have a clearer mind, sort out our thoughts and emotions, making our communication more productive both at work and in social life. We can focus more easily and accordingly feel less stressed. We become more aware of our emotions; hence, we can manage them more effectively. We find a solution sooner in areas of our lives where we feel stuck. It promotes the processing of mental problems. It helps to find peace and balance. We get closer to understanding ourselves, the people around us, our lives, and our mission. When we accept ourselves as we are, we become positive, joyful, and attractive. This will make our existing relationship more intimate or, if we are alone, the desired partner will come into our lives.

The Power of Affirmation

Our affirmations are nothing more than repeated statements in a given situation, whereby we comment on the pleasant or unpleasant effects of that situation inside us. If you observe these inner comments, you will find that they are repetitive elements that we happen to say very often to ourselves. However, we don't pay enough attention to selecting them and therefore, they can be either positive or negative. In fact, the very source of our low self-esteem is that we tend to repeat more negative affirmations than positive ones. Have you ever happened to say these sentences to yourself: "I can't do that"; "It won't work anyway"; "I have no power over it"; "They're better than me anyway"?

We need to know, that like every word, every thought has a certain level and degree of energy. Since an uttered word represents higher and more powerful energy than thought, every statement has a very significant energy content. Negative statements, by their very nature, carry negative energy, so their regular repetition results in the feeding of negative energies. Positive statements, on the other hand, are saturated with positive energy content, so if they are repeated systematically, we can reach positive energy multiplication. Positive affirmations are statements that describe the purpose we want to accomplish. These sentences, if repeated often, stimulate our minds. That's why it's essential to program your brain with positive affirmations. Our subconscious mind follows exactly what we say to it, because it takes our words as commands. Give your brain positive instructions, so that you will have a more successful life.

With the proper saturation of thought energy, the thought can materialize (come to fruition), whether positive or negative. A very good example is how Bonnie used to reject the offer of delicious food by saying, "I can't take it because of my eating problems!" As long she had such - surely negative - statements (about her overweight state), she indeed remained overweight. To make matters worse, by saying that one specific food makes us gain weight, we don't do anything other than put its name into the "fattening" category, and as a result of this negative programming, we will indeed gain weight.

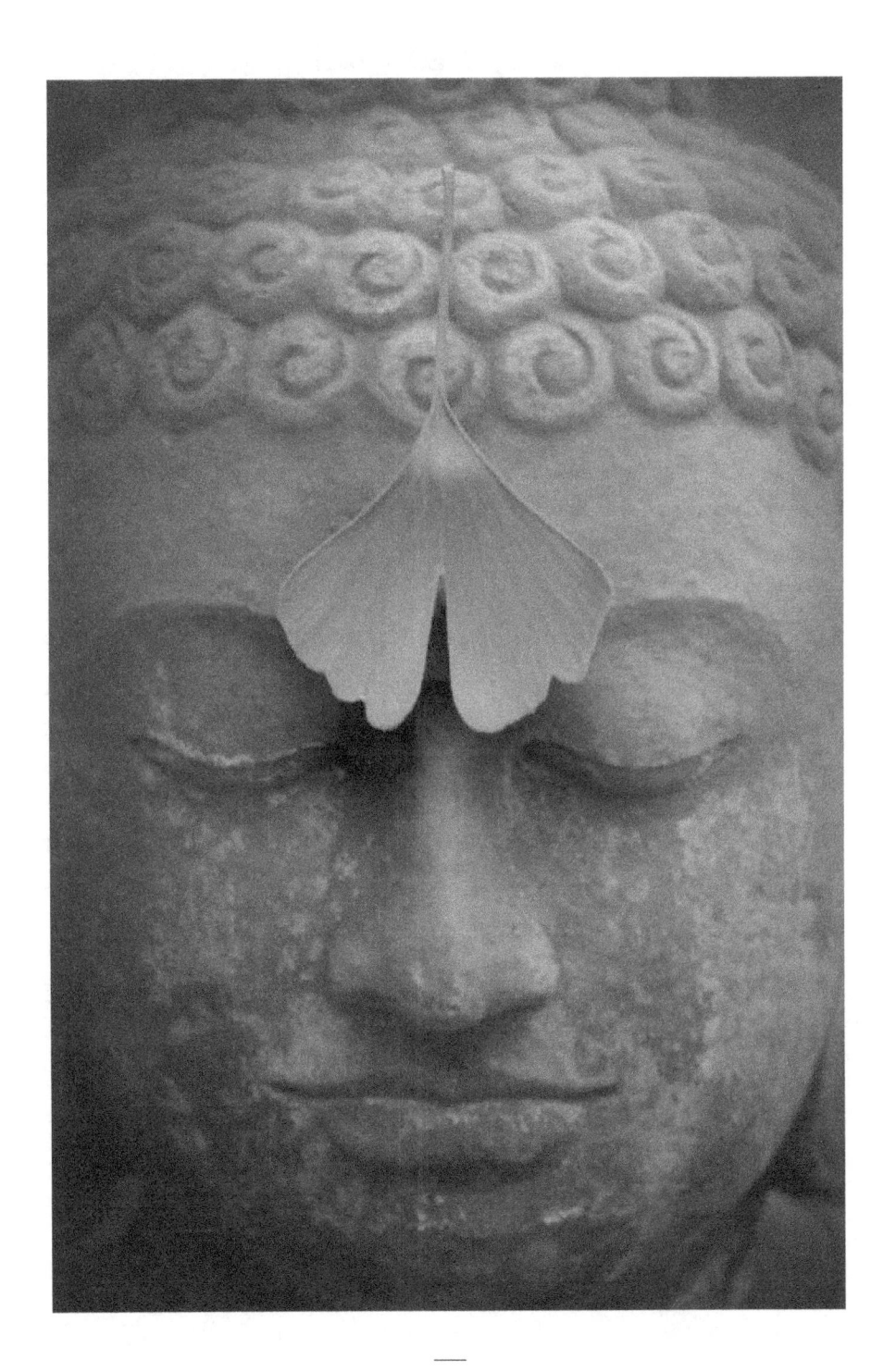

Why Meditate?

What are the Benefits of Meditation?

The reasons we meditate are as varied as the numerous ways there are to meditate. In the West, the vast majority are attracted to reflection to calm the interior babble of the mind and to lessen pressure. Reflection is, undoubtedly, a successful pressure reducer, however its advantages—here and there strangely covered up—are unquestionably increasingly abundant.

The genuine demonstration of contemplation can be as basic as sitting unobtrusively and concentrating on your breath or a mantra—a word or expression. There are endless conventions and no particular "right" approach to rehearsing reflection. Discover training that you like and stick with it for some time. Notice how you feel as you approach your days. On the off chance that you find that you have more tolerance, feel grounded and better ready to react to unpleasant circumstances, and are more in contact with your instinct or "hunches," you are getting a charge out of the numerous advantages of reflection.

It is Good for Our Bodies

Researchers gathering information on reflection have discovered that a steady practice helps the brain; however, it likewise reinforces the body. Studies confirm that reflection can help turn around coronary illness, decrease torment, and bolster the invulnerable framework, better empowering it to battle malady.

The mind-body association between stress and illness is copiously clear as science is finding that contemplation can bring down the generation of the pressure hormone cortisol. This implies meditators are better ready to adjust to worry in their lives and its normal physiologic reactions, which can include:

- Coronary illness
- Osteoporosis
- Rest issues
- Stomach related issues
- Gloom
- Heftiness
- Memory weakness
- Skin conditions

Because It's Good for Our Relationships

Incomprehensibly, while reflection causes us to tune in and go internal to our actual pith, it likewise encourages us to separate from our own self-images to associate with others in increasingly important manners. Couples advisors have discovered when they allocate their customers contemplation, the couples become less irate, increasingly self-intelligent, and all the more cherishing.

When we become mindful of—and respect—our interconnection with different creatures, we can recast our points of view, see our stresses from an alternate perspective, and grasp appreciation, which is the heart's memory.

Because it can Change Our Lives

In a world overflowing with ceaseless quick fixes, crash eats less, and pyramid schemes, it's pleasant to know there is a demonstrated practice that truly can transform you (or if nothing else achieve emotional impacts) in only a brief period in every day.

Yogis and specialists both concur – thinking — even only a couple of minutes of profound breathing—loosens up the mind, diminishes tension, and diminishes discouragement. When we feel like we cannot bear the cost of an opportunity to meditate, however in all actuality we cannot manage the cost of not to.

Myths Behind Meditation

Meditation is profoundly close to personal practice. When you have built up training that works for you, odds are that you will keep on sharpening that training until you see its advantages pervading your life. You are probably going to feel increasingly adjusted, not so much pushed, but rather more present and mindful. In the beginning times of our training, be that as it may, a significant number of us feel stuck, attempting to get it without flaw.

There is nobody approach to "hit the nail on the head," and there are some regular fantasies and misguided judgments about contemplation that may thwart you from advancing as easily or as fast as you would like. Here is a couple:

1. There is just a single method to contemplate.

On the off chance that there was just a single method to ponder, contemplation would not be so far-reaching all things considered. In fact, there are various styles and systems of reflection to look over.

For instance, there is open checking reflection (where the focal point of contemplation is simply the experience, as opposed to a specific article), and centered mindfulness contemplation (with the center coordinated toward a particular item, for example, the breath or a mantra).

Search for a style of reflection that impacts you, regardless of whether it's strolling contemplation, innovative contemplation (envisioning and fortifying positive parts of the psyche), lovingkindness contemplation (broadening sentiments of adoration and empathy toward others), or some other style that addresses you. There is such a large number to pick from!

Be that as it may, remember to look for direction from an educator who can enable you to take advantage of the maximum capacity of reflective practice. Converse with individual yogis and check whether they can suggest a decent contemplation instructor, or search for an educator on the web. Maybe you as of now have a yoga educator who can offer you knowledge into reflection. Get inquisitive, and do not be reluctant to pose inquiries. Contemplation—in any structure—requires the professional's truthfulness and hence will include some examination on your part.

2. You need to discharge your psyche to Meditate.

Ask anybody on the road what they think contemplation includes, and you'll most likely get depictions of somebody sitting leg over the leg in a dim room, palms up, with thumbs and index fingers contacting, reciting OM. You will additionally likely hear that an objective of contemplation is to "void your brain." This is not exact. Individuals endeavoring to discharge their brains are frequently defeated on the grounds that our psyches are once in a while very still. Does this mean contemplation is worthless? Obviously not. The key is not to obstruct our considerations or void our psyche, yet rather to enable each idea to travel in complete disorder.

Everybody will have musings during reflection, and a few contemplations will be totally disconnected from your training. Yet, reflecting—regardless of the style—is a chance to prepare the psyche so as not to wind up assimilated in those considerations. For instance, in case you are rehearsing open observing reflection, your activity, as a meditator will be to recognize the contemplations you have, be with them, and enable them to go through you. In centered mindfulness reflection, you will draw your consideration, over and over, back to the object of center (a mantra or your breath). What's more, when diverting contemplations enter, you recognize them and enable them to pass, as opposed to attempting to smother them or push them away.

3. To meditate, you need to sit for quite a long time at once.

A few experts think for quite a long time at once (this is standard practice at Vipassana withdraws, for instance). In any case, while their dedication is excellent, even fortunate, such length in contemplation basically is not attainable for the greater part of us regularly. What's more, the commonness of the legend that so as to ponder you should devote hours, leads numerous potential specialists to accept they basically do not have adequate time.

Luckily, reflection does not need to expend an excessive amount of time. Similarly, as there are numerous styles of reflection, there are numerous approaches to fit it into your day by day life. When you pick a style of reflection that works for you, you can likewise measure to what extent rehearsing that style works for you. Possibly ten minutes daily is best for your calendar, or perhaps less. You likewise do not need to hop directly in. Arrangement for training is similarly significant, and it does not need to be massively tedious. You can utilize something as basic as breathing activities, which can be as short as three to five minutes. In any case, while the length of contemplation and its arrangement do not should be too much longer, you do need to make a responsibility. It is commonly increasingly helpful to rehearse routinely for a short measure of time than to rehearse for a more drawn out time sporadically. You will benefit from your training by transforming it into a propensity.

4. Quick outcomes.

Numerous individuals go into reflection searching for snappy outcomes. While the facts confirm that reflection can lead specialists into significant conditions of internal harmony, do not expect such outcomes right away. Reflection is not simple. It requires some investment to wind up familiar with it and to receive the rewards of training.

Individuals who concentrate the specialty of contemplation may rehearse for a considerable length of time before they make huge leaps forward. Reflection sets aside some effort to ace. In spite of the fact that ruminating may look straightforward from the outset, the measure of mental and otherworldly development required so as to get to more profound conditions of internal harmony is frequently tremendous.

Gaining ground in contemplation requires practice and persistence. Consider it something you are building. Numerous basic and apparently monotonous advances go into setting up the establishment, all basic to the structure's strength. Skirt one corner, or forget about a post, and at some point, or another it could all wind up shaky. In the event that you do not verify the establishment, your training may correspondingly self-destruct, and you may well surrender it.

Setting aside the effort to construct a strong establishment by concentrating on the fundamentals guarantees that you become entrenched before proceeding onward to the subsequent stage.

5. Meditation is a Strict Religious practice.

For some individuals, contemplation may sound awkwardly strict. All that discussion about otherworldliness and self-acknowledgment can be scary and may even divert one's attention from reflection. While contemplation can be otherworldly, and it is available in various world religions, for example, Jainism, Buddhism, Hinduism, and even Christianity—you do not need to be strict or profoundly centered to rehearse it.

Contemplation is definitely not a closed-minded practice. The act of reflection just involves various techniques for reconnecting you to your deepest self. Contemplation can be a simple common action too.

In spite of the fact that the language of reflective practices may now and again use strict terminology (with terms, for example, "nirvana," "chakra," or "kundalini"), please keep in mind that it is simple language. The jargon is as rich as ever, and these words are utilized to convey inner encounters or vibes of certain specialists. In any case, these are encounters that could conceivably concern you—and that is all right!

Understanding the history of meditation is important to debunk the myths surrounding the practice. You have learned about a few forms of meditation practice. However, there are numerous ways one can practice meditation as long as it works for you. Meditation practice seems to be surrounded by mystery hence creating various myths. However, we believe with the discussion here, you will be able to debunk the myths and embrace this practice as you benefit from it.

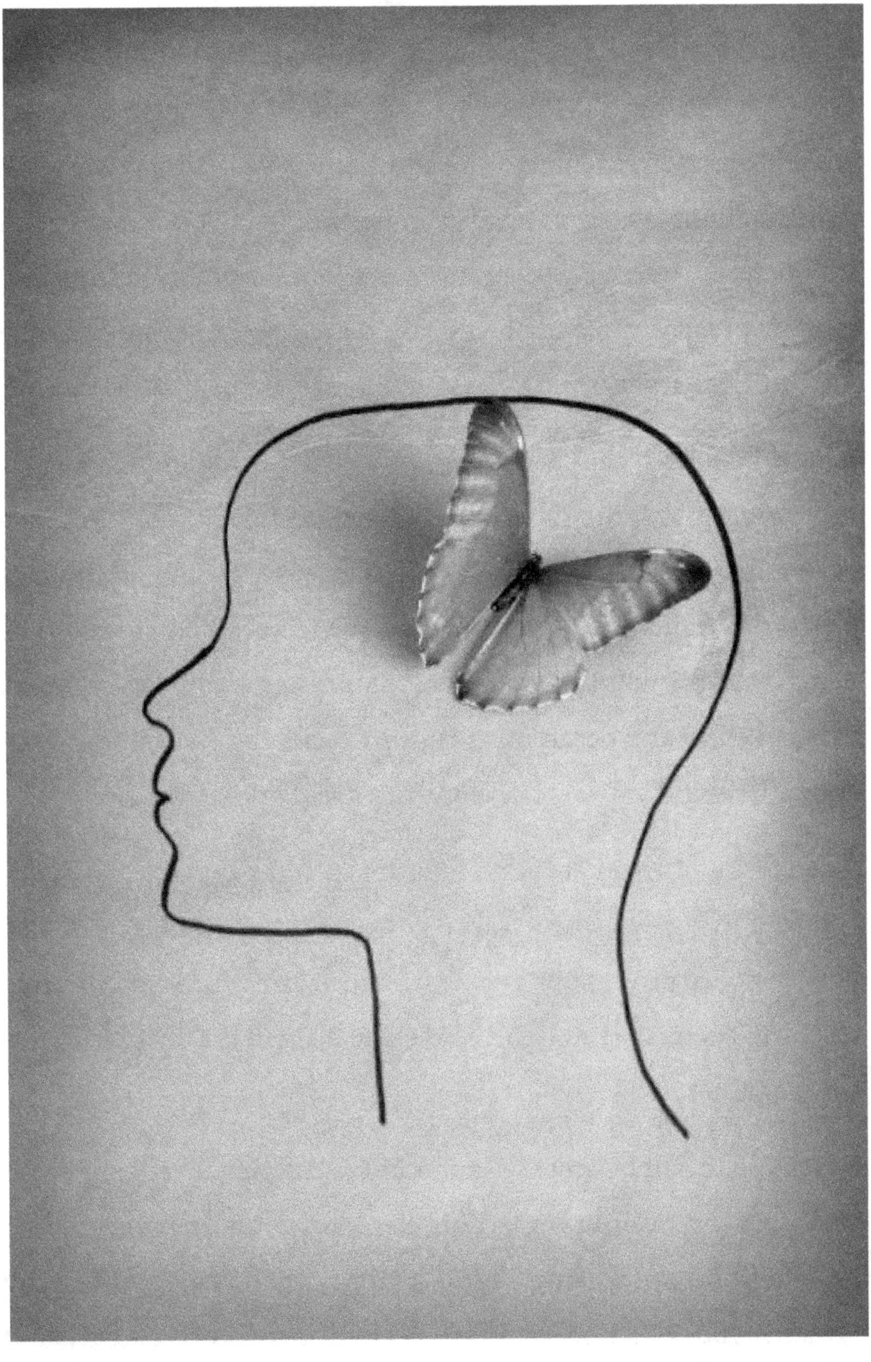

What Is Being Mindful?

The concept of mindfulness was first researched in the 1970s by psychologists and, to this day, it is one of the most intensely studied areas of psychology. Mindfulness is very simply bringing your thoughts back to the present moment so that you are experiencing what is happening in the here-and-now, as opposed to your present moment being colored by apprehensions of the future or concerns over the past.

Mindfulness as a skill is not just a good self-development tool. It can be very helpful in the workplace and even vital in some careers. A centered and sharp focus is vital to jobs like police officers, paramedics, emergency room doctors and firefighters. Being able to maintain focus in the present moment can be a matter of life and death for people in such jobs and certainly for you too, should you be on the receiving end of their services.

It can be helpful in parenting in order to allow us to focus on our children in that moment and enjoy them. Mindfulness can also help us not to project our own fears and desires onto our children, allowing them to simply be who they are and not images of our own making.

Mindfulness can be an excellent tool in studying. Every time you shift your attention to something else, your brain burns glucose to do so. If you are attempting to study without being mindfully present, you will find that you become tired very quickly and struggle to retain the information that you have studied in that session. By being mindful, your brain only has to focus on the task at hand and all your energy can be employed in that task.

Benefits of Mindfulness for Your Body

One body. That is all you're going to get in this lifetime. That's all everyone is going to get. One life, one body, one mind, heart, and soul. If you don't cherish the body that you have and take care of it the way it deserves, it won't be long before your body starts to break down gradually. You won't even feel it at first or realize that it is happening until it's too late to do anything about it. Your body is the vehicle that you are going to journey through life with, and you must take care of it both on the inside and out for better health physically, emotionally, and mentally.

Mindfulness is one of the many ways in which you will come to realize what your body needs and what it does not, and it certainly does not need the stress that you put it through every day. Actively practicing mindfulness brings awareness to just how much your body is affected by stress, especially when it manifests itself as physical pain. We've covered some of the basic reasons why mindfulness is good for you in general, but now let's focus on what it can do specifically for your body.

Bringing awareness to the way that your body feels through each experience will help you forge a closer connection to your body in a way that you never have before. By frequently "scanning" your body for an overall assessment of how you feel, you start to notice all the little things that you missed before you began practicing mindfulness. You notice every itch, every ache, and every tingle even in the smallest parts of your body. You notice when you start to feel any pain in your body, you notice when you feel cold, warm, pleasantly comfortable, and more. All of the sensations that you feel will always be accompanied by some emotion or thought, and it is through mindfulness that you start to listen to what your body is trying to tell you.

Benefit #1 - Possible Slowdown of Aging Cells. Who wouldn't want to look younger if they could? The beauty industry is a booming business for one simple reason. We're always on the lookout for the proverbial fountain of youth. Anything that holds the promise of turning back the clock and reversing the signs of aging gives us a little bit of hope. Yet, the easiest way to slow down the signs of aging, as it turns out, could be to practice mindfulness to minimize stress. Cell aging is a natural occurrence, but it is sped up by stress, unhealthy lifestyle choices, and the diseases we contract. Some studies suggest that those who practice long-term mindfulness meditation could potentially have greater telomere lengths. Telomeres are a protein that is at the end of the chromosomes in our bodies. This protein is the one responsible for protecting our chromosomes from the signs of aging, and it would seem mindfulness has a positive impact on this. That would explain why some scientists appear to be optimistic that mindfulness could be the anti-aging fountain of youth we've been searching high and low for all along.

Benefit #2 - Better Heart Health. It's no secret that heart disease is one of the leading causes of death, especially in the United States, with one in four deaths annually attributed to this condition. Given that heart disease is associated with chronic stress levels, mindfulness is the way towards better heart health, given the circumstances. In a study that was conducted on participants who were dealing with pre-hypertension, those who learned how to meditate mindfully showed significantly greater improvements in their diastolic and systolic blood pressure levels. This was in comparison to other participants who were given an augmented drug as their treatment instead of a mindfulness program. This suggests that mindfulness could have an important role to play in lowering the risk of high blood pressure and the associated heart conditions that go along with it. Yet another study that was conducted revealed that participants who chose to undergo a mindfulness program had a significant improvement in their 6-minute walking test that measured their cardiovascular capacity.

Benefit #3 - A Healthy Pathway to Weight Management. Weight gain or weight loss are some of the many symptoms associated with excessive stress. Yet, we brush it off and don't think twice about the connection between these symptoms and stress. We don't realize how this behavior pattern and way of thinking of is having damaging effects on our health. When you're preoccupied with stress, there are two ways you could react to it. One, you'll eat in excess as a coping mechanism to feel better, which will result in weight gain. Two, the stress you feel could be so intense that you lose your appetite entirely. Neither approach is healthy, and without mindfulness, it's going to be hard to break out of this destructive cycle. Living in a world today that is designed for convenience certainly isn't helping matters, with fast food and deep-fried unhealthy options available around every corner. The only way to put a stop to it is through mindful awareness. To realize why you feel the way you do, what's causing it, how you're reacting towards it, and what you need to do to put a stop to it.

Benefit #4 - Promotes Better Sleep. It is amazing what a good night's sleep can do for you. Yet, struggling with insomnia and poor, restless sleep at night is becoming an all too common phenomenon these days. Especially when our minds are riddled with worries. How many times have you found yourself lying in bed awake at night, tossing and turning as you tried to get some sleep, yet all you could think about was how stressed you feel? Every day, our lives present us with new challenges. Every day, we try to find a balance between managing our careers, families, relationships, finances, health, and wellbeing. By the time the end of the day approaches, you feel so exhausted, drained of energy that you go through the motions without connecting with the world around you. Excessive worry is going to have both long and short-term effects on your wellbeing. Not getting enough sleep will affect your ability to make decisions, rob you of happiness, and aggravate any physical medical conditions you already have, which are often associated with high levels of stress. You need mindfulness for better sleep at night; it will do your body a world of good.

Benefit #5 - Greater Resilience, Physically and Mentally. Mindfulness is about bettering yourself overall, and it encompasses several aspects that go beyond learning how to control your thoughts. One of these aspects involves building resilience, both mentally and physically, to overcome the obstacles and challenges that are thrown your way. There are only two ways to achieve the goals you set for yourself - one is to set them, two is to achieve them. Most of the time, when we give up and feel physically unable to push forward anymore, it is often because our mind has given up first. Without resilience, the desire to give up can be too overwhelming to reject. Setbacks, failures, disappointments along the way, feeling like every time you take one step forward, you take two steps back, that is enough to wear you down and can diminish the desire that you have to keep on pushing forward. When stress becomes a byproduct of these emotions, your body starts to feel defeated as the symptoms begin manifesting physically in the form of aches, pains, and muscular tension. It won't be long before you eventually give up altogether because it does not seem worth it to keep going anymore.

Benefit #6 - Coping Mechanism for Depression. Depression is one of the most debilitating mental conditions that a person can experience. Depression robs you of joy and makes life feel like it is a constant struggle. Feelings of despair, hopelessness, and unhappiness that cannot be explained threaten to drown you in what may seem to be a never-ending cycle of misery. Some days you don't even feel like you have the energy to get out of bed because depression can be so overwhelming. Sometimes it feels like there is nothing that can help you, and it is exactly why you need mindfulness. It has been used for centuries to achieve mental well-being and happiness, satisfaction, emotional stability. When combined with mindfulness meditation, it reduces and minimizes the risk of experiencing depression by limiting the production of excess cortisol in your body, which has been known to be the cause of many stress-related disorders, depression included. Both mindfulness and meditation are effective in helping you balance the neurotransmitters in your brain, especially dopamine and serotonin, which have been strongly linked to causing depression.

Benefit #7 - It Allows Greater Control Over Your Emotions. Our emotions are sensitive to what is happening around us. When you're stressed, you're emotional. Emotions can get the best of you when you don't know how to control them. This is why learning to slow down your thoughts and emotions deliberately can go a long way towards helping you learn how to exercise greater self-regulation over your actions. Being emotional can make it difficult to keep a clear head, and you react based on your impulses instead. Mindfulness helps you stay in control every step of the way, so you are the one who remains in the driver's seat always.

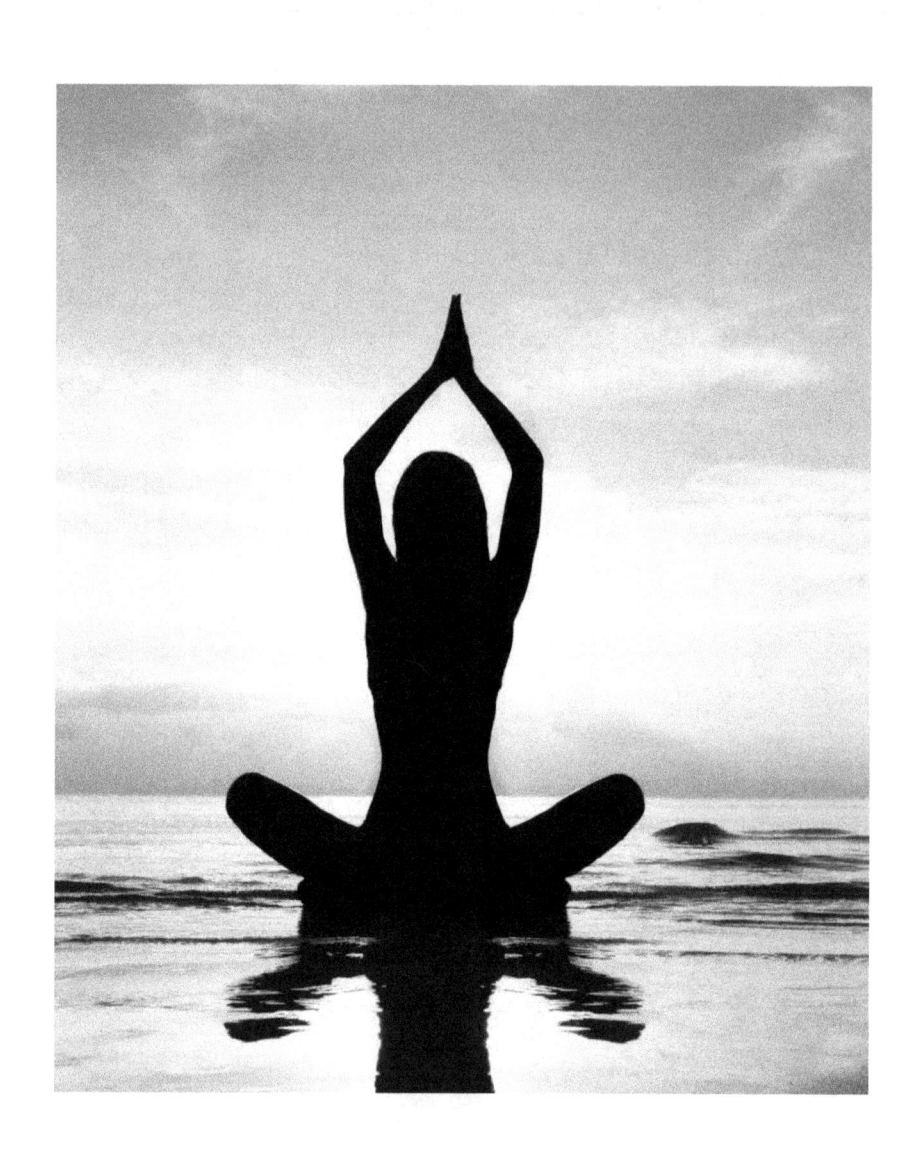

Starting Your Meditation Journey

Meditation Techniques You Can Use

Mantra Meditation

This is a type of meditation designed to encourage peace, love, and unity, and cultivate and strengthen a sense of compassion. This technique is especially useful if you're having trouble with relationships, or if people are the source of your stress.

1. This meditation works with any position you're comfortable with. Start by practicing breathing meditation for a minute or two. Start focusing on yourself and use positive mantras to send your goodwill towards yourself. Here are some examples of positive mantras:

- let me be safe

- let me be calm

- let me be happy

- let me find peace

You can use as many mantras as you want, and it's up to you whether you say them out loud or just in your head.

2. Keep meditating on yourself for a minute or so. Then, imagine someone you care about, like a lover, a friend, or a family

member. Use similar mantras to wish them well and send out your affection and goodwill.

3. After meditating on a loved one for a few minutes, turn your focus to someone for whom you don't have strong feelings, positive or negative, and send them your feelings of compassion or goodwill.

4. The last step is always the most difficult. Visualize someone you have negative feelings for, be it a coworker who rubs you the wrong way, the drunk driver who almost crashed into you on your way home, a group of people whose way of doing things you strongly disagree with, or even the stray cat that sneaks into your house at night and leaves a big mess everywhere. Meditate on them and use mantras to help you declare feelings of compassion and goodwill for them too. These feelings may not be very genuine at the start, but with repeated practice, that may change.

This type of meditation can bring up strong emotions when visualizing someone you like or someone you don't like. While you shouldn't try to reject those emotions and try to push them away, you shouldn't invite them or dwell on them either. Focus purely on your mantra and the feelings of compassion, unity, and goodwill that you are trying to project.

Body Scan Meditation

This is a form of meditation that focuses on getting to know your body and making sure to relax every part of it.

This meditation is also suitable for any meditation position, but many believe that lying down works best.

1. Spend a minute meditating on your breathing, then turn your focus to your feet. Try to identify all the sensations you can feel in your feet. If you notice any discomfort or tension, try to relieve it. A good way to do this is to imagine breathing air into your feet and letting your muscles slacken.

2. Once your feet are done, move on to your legs. Repeat the process of identifying sensations and relaxing your legs. Keep doing this, gradually moving up your body until you've reached your head. For a short session, you can break your body into fairly large parts, like feet, legs, back, chest arms, hands, shoulders, neck, head. Or you can make it a longer session by doing a more refined scan - toes, feet, ankles, calves, knees, thighs, etc. Make sure you spend extra time on parts of your body that have been under a lot of strain or causing pain recently.

3. Once you've reached your head, meditate on your breathing again for a short while.

4. Repeat the whole process of scanning your body in reverse, starting with your head and moving down to your toes.

Chakra Meditation

Chakras are an important element in managing the flow of energy and are believed to be the points where energy enters the body and is distributed to the rest of your limbs. There are seven chakras in the body located along the spine, directly over the main nerve centers of the nervous system. Each chakra has a specific function and is influenced by related elements in your life. The seven chakras are also each associated with a color, and a mudra and mantra used when meditating. Meditation can be used to open and strengthen the chakras.

First is the Root chakra. It is located at the base of the spine and deals with your natural survival instinct and basic needs. It is blocked by fear and insecurity. The root chakra is associated with the color red, and its mantra during meditation is LAM. Its mudra is the Jnana.

Second is the Sacral chakra, which is located just beneath the naval and manages your reproductive capabilities and all creative elements of the mind. It's associated with the color orange and uses the VAM chakra. For its mudra, rest your hands in your lap with your right hand on top of the left and both palms facing upward. Lift your thumbs and bring the tips together to form a rough circle.

The third chakra is the Solar Plexus chakra and is located directly on top of your belly button. This chakra focuses on both physical and mental power and is important in accepting new experiences. It also helps with digestion. The associated color is yellow, and the mantra is RAM. For the mudra, bring your hands together in front of you between your chest and stomach. Cross your thumbs and turn your hands so your fingertips face forward.

Fourth is the Heart chakra, which is located in the center of your chest. It's strongly connected to your heart and deals with emotions, specifically feelings of love and affection, and healing. The mantra is YAM, the color is green, and for the mudra you use the Jnana, but rather than resting on your knee, your right hand is held over the physical location of the chakra.

Fifth is the Throat chakra which is located in the throat and deals with honesty and communication. It's associated with the color blue and uses the HAM mantra. The mudra is similar to the one used with the Sacral chakra, but rather than resting your hands-on top of each other to form a bigger, more exact circle.

The sixth chakra is the Third-Eye chakra. It is located in the center of your forehead, and deals with intuition and understanding, both mundane and spiritual. It is also believed to be connected to psychic abilities. It is represented by the color purple and uses the

SHANG mantra. For the mudra, bring your hands together in front of your chest. Bend all your fingers except the middle fingers and thumbs down at the first joint and press them to their counterpart on the opposite hand. Straighten your middle fingers and press their tips together. Relax your thumbs.

Weight Loss, Meditation and Mindset: How They're Linked to Each Other

Contemplation can be a perception that connects the brain and body to a method for quieting. Individuals have been pondering as a non-mainstream perception for a large number of years. Today, a considerable lot of us are utilizing reflection to decrease pressure and get a great deal of checking out their contemplations. There are numerous sorts of contemplation estimated in a square. The utilization of explicit expressions known as mantras was bolstered by some square measure. Others center around breathing or keeping the brain in the present. Every one of these ways will enable you to build up a vastly improved comprehension of yourself, yet your brain and body cooperate.

This expanded mindfulness makes reflection a helpful device to comprehend your dietary patterns better, which could prompt weight reduction. Peruse on to become familiar with the weight reduction advantages of reflection and how to begin.

What are the advantages of weight loss meditation?

Continued weight reduction

Contemplation won't make you get in shape medium-term. In any case, with a little practice, it might have enduring impacts on your weight, yet additionally on your examples of reasoning. Contemplation is related to an assortment of advantages.

Mindfulness contemplation is, by all accounts, the most accommodating as far as weight reduction. A survey of existing examinations in 2017 found that reflection on cognizance was a compelling method to get in shape and change dietary patterns.

Reflection of care includes giving close consideration to where are you, and are you doing what you feel right now? All through the contemplation of care, you will perceive every one of these perspectives without judgment. Attempt to regard your contemplations and activities as those by themselves—nothing else. Consider what you feel and do, yet don't attempt to group anything as positive or negative. Standard practice makes this simpler.

Rehearsing reflection with mindfulness can likewise bring about long-term benefits. As per a 2017 survey, the individuals who practice mindfulness are bound to keep the weight off contrasted with different health food nuts.

Less blame and disgrace

Contemplation of care can be particularly helpful in checking passionate and stress-related eating. You can perceive those occasions when you eat because you are pushed, instead of hungry, by ending up progressively mindful of your considerations and feelings.

It is additionally a decent instrument to keep you from falling into the unsafe winding of disgrace and blame for which a few people fall when they attempt to change their dietary patterns. Contemplation caution includes recognizing your sentiments and practices for what they are, without deciding for you.

How might I start to mull overweight reduction? Reflection can be polished by anybody with the psyche and body. No extraordinary gear or costly classes are required. For some, finding the time is the hardest part. Attempt to begin with a sensible thing, similar to 10 minutes per day or even every other day.

Ensure that during these 10 minutes, you approach a tranquil spot. You might need to crush it in on the off chance that you have children before they wake up or after they hit the sack to limit diversion. In the shower, you can even attempt to do it.

Make yourself agreeable once you are in a tranquil spot. In any position that feels simple, you can sit or rest. Start by concentrating on your breath, watching the ascent and fall of your chest or stomach. Feel the air moving all through your nose or mouth. Hear the sounds that the air makes. Do these for a couple of minutes until you feel increasingly loose?

Please follow these steps with your eyes open or shut:

- Take a full breath in.

- Keep it for a couple of moments.

- Exhale gradually and rehash.

Breathe.

- Observe your breath as it streams into your noses, raises your chest, or moves your midsection, however not the slightest bit modify it.

- Continue centering for 5 to 10 minutes on your breath.

- You're going to discover your mind, meandering, which is very ordinary. Simply perceive that your psyche has meandered and taken your consideration back to your breath.

- Reflect on how effectively your brain meandered as you wrap up. Perceive then that it was so natural to reestablish your regard for your breath.

Attempt to accomplish a larger number of weekdays than not. Remember that in an initial couple of times you do, it may not feel exceptionally effective. Be that as it may, it will end up less complex with successive exercise and start to feel progressively regular.

The Power of Repeated Words and Thoughts

Recollect how you used to rehash something again and again so as to retain it for a test? At the point when done over some stretch of time, rehashed words and contemplations will in general become lasting. By rehashing your insistences, your brain will gradually surrender and Believe what you're letting yourself know.

Reinventing the Subconscious Mind

The psyche mind is the most remarkable piece of our cerebrum, but at the same time it's the hardest to control. Inside the inner mind, the entirety of your actual expectations, dreams, fears, and bad dreams are put away.

The motivation behind why a few insistences don't work is that the psyche mind has not been persuaded and is consequently as yet pulling in negative occasions. All together for your insistences to begin producing results throughout your life, you need to fool the inner mind into tolerating your certifications.

Here are a few hints to enable your confirmations to break through to your inner mind:

Discover the harmony among aspiring and reasonable – many individuals go over the edge with their confirmations. A few people who are gaining a no and are covered in the red may attempt to state, "I am rich, and I win $100,000 every month." obviously, the inner mind knows immediately this isn't accurate. One approach to fix this isn't really to mitigate the fantasy, yet to include more authenticity into it, e.g., "I have the quality and assurance to liberate myself from obligations and work harder to procure $100,000 every month."

Give your inner mind confirmation that your assertions are valid – insistence alone won't transform you; you need to blend in real life also. Confirmations like "I have a strong constitution" are pointless if not joined with appropriate exercise, rest, and sustenance. A superior variant of the past insistence would be: "I decide to practice in any event three times each week, get at any rate 7 hours of rest, and eat well food in light of the fact that my strong physical make-up is on its way."

Make certifications that inspire forceful feelings – notice how many individuals recall effectively occasions that made them cry, chuckle, and so on. Ensure that when you make confirmations, you incorporate descriptive words that bring out cheerful, moving and inspirational considerations. Rather than saying "I decide to get up early every morning," state, "I decide to get up early every early daytime feeling energized, revived, and prepared to take on the day!"

Ensure your assertion targets you – tailor your insistences particularly for yourself. For instance, an attestation like "My supervisor will give me an advancement" is somewhat frail since that assertion focuses on your chief and not yourself; you don't have any power over your chief. Rather, settle on something like "I decide to feel that I generally get quality work turned in and thusly merit an advancement."

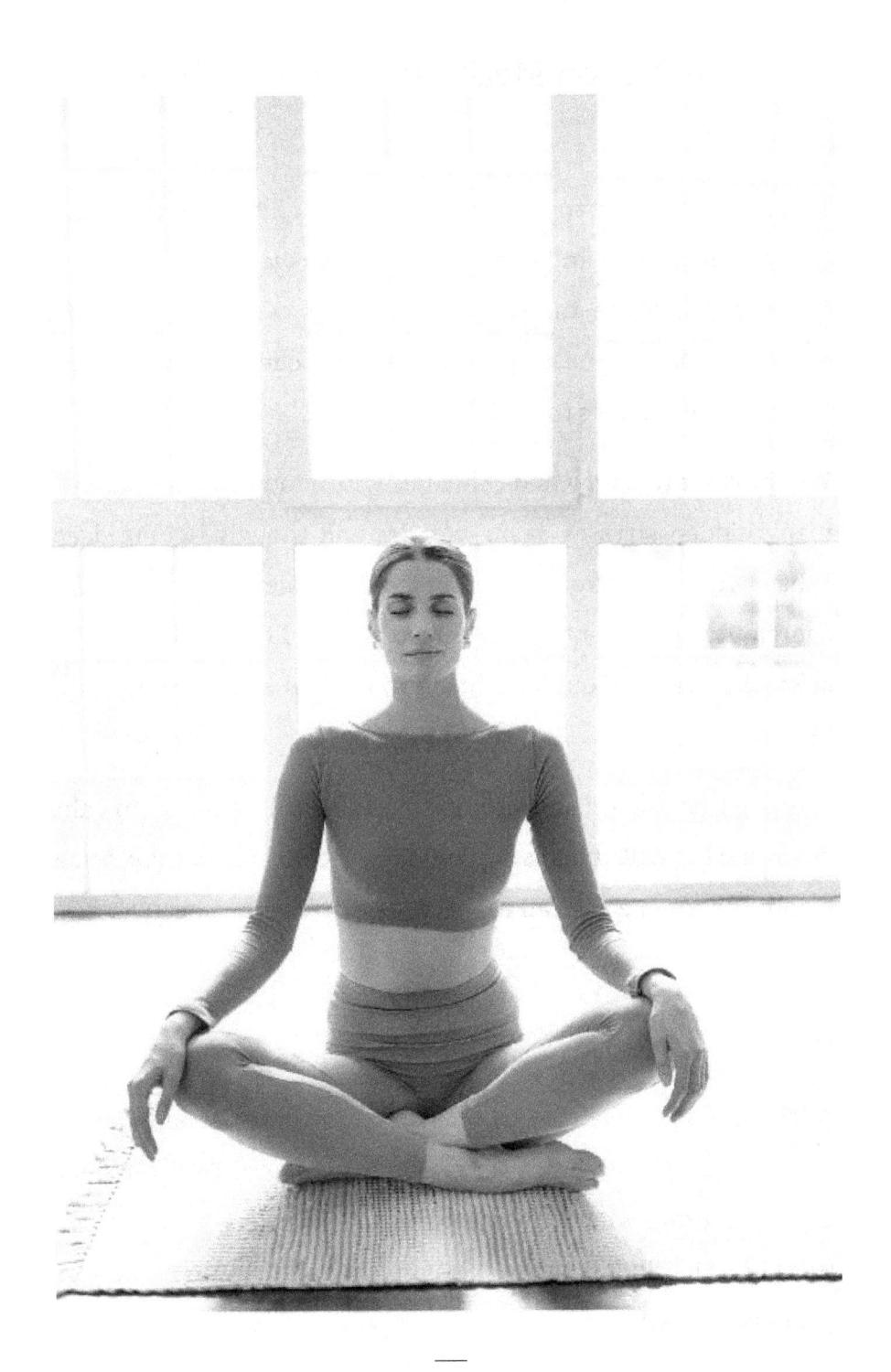

Meditation Methods to Lose Weight

Today's world is just so fast-paced that it feels like we have no time to slow down, relax and be calm. Even when we go on holiday, we take over the office and work in our heads, worrying about the succeeding board meeting, a disgruntled client, or where the following deal comes from.

We think we're happy and calm, but within our minds, there are many hidden stresses, fears, worries and thoughts going deep. When we don't take time to relax and quiet the inner noise consciously and intentionally, tension will build up and inevitably affect the quality of our lives, and how we deal with people around us.

It needn't be like this. Meditation practice will allow us to calm down and get still. It helps our mind to get concentrated and relax, helping us to cope with all the everyday stresses of a hectic life.

Meditative Advantages.

A lot of people have various reasons to meditate. When you are contemplating, what was your reason to meditate? To an outsider, if you meditate what they see you do is sit down, maybe cross-legged on the floor, staring at a point in the distance or sit with your eyes closed.

Meditation is some mental activity that has significant health benefits both for the mind and the body. Meditation can help relax the mind, establish a more concentrated state and enhance the functioning of the brain.

Methods of meditation

Conscious Meditation. It's easy to get caught up in a loop of spinning thoughts — starting to think about a laundry list of activities to do, ruminating about past events, or potentially future situations — and practicing mindfulness may help. Yet what exactly is attention? It can be described as a mental state that requires being fully engaged on "the now" so that, without judgment, you can understand and acknowledge your thoughts, feelings and sensations.

Mindfulness meditation is a form of mental preparation that helps you to slow down thoughts of running, let go of anger and relax both your mind and body. Mindfulness methods can vary, but a meditation on mindfulness generally involves breathing exercise, mental imagery, body and mind awareness, and relaxation of the muscle and organ. Practicing meditation with mindfulness does not require props or planning (no need for candles, essential oils or mantras, unless you enjoy it). To get going, all you need is a comfortable sitting spot, three to five minutes of spare time and an attitude that's free of judgment.

Mindfulness meditation is the method of having your thoughts fully present. Knowledge involves being mindful of where we are and what we do, and not being too sensitive to what is happening around us.

One can do reflective meditation anywhere. Some people like to sit in a quiet spot, close their eyes and focus on their respiration. But at every stage of the day, even when driving to work or doing chores, you can choose to be conscious.

You track your thoughts and feelings while practicing mindfulness meditation but let them move without judgment.

Transcendental meditation. Transcendental meditation is an essential technique whereby an individually defined rhythm, such as a word, sound, or short phrase, is repeated in a particular way. It is exercised twice per day for 20 minutes while sitting comfortably close to the eyes.

The hope is that this technique will allow you to settle into a deep state of relaxation to achieve inner peace without attention or effort.

Directed Meditation. Directed meditation, often also referred to as guided imagery or visualization, is a meditation technique in which you create mental images or scenarios that you find calming.

Vipassana Meditation. Vipassana meditation is an ancient form of Indian meditation which means seeing things as they are. More than 2,500 years ago, it was taught in India. Conscious meditation movement has origins in this practice in the United States.

The purpose of meditation with vipassana is self-transformation through the examination of oneself. The sustained interconnectedness leads to a happy account filled with love and compassion.

Vipassana is usually taught during a 10-day course in this tradition, and people are expected to follow a set of rules all the time, as well as for abstaining from all intoxicants, telling lies, cheating, sexual activity, and killing any animals.

Meditation Yoga. The yoga practice has its roots in ancient India. There are a wide variety of yoga classes and styles, but all include performing a series of postures and guided breathing exercises designed to encourage flexibility and relax the mind.

The poses require balance and attention, and practitioners are encouraged to concentrate less on distractions and remain more at the moment.

Which meditation style you choose to try, depends on several factors. When you have a health problem and are new to yoga, tell your doctor what method would be right for you.

Ways to Promote Meditation into Your Life.

Treat yourself to ice cream? Are you stuck in the motorway? A friend in wait? Here's how to make these moments a meditation.

Which one considers harder: in sleep, taming your monkey mind or making extra time only to sit still every day? Either way, fear not: by merely integrating meditation into your daily activities, you can quickly reach a calm state of mind.

Do that you want to do. If it's hiking, walking, cooking or painting, while we concentrate wholeheartedly on our favorite things, time stands still. Mysteriously, our stream of emotions, stories and dramas fall away. Submerge yourself in this One Amazing Thing, and don't pay heed to those pings! Then keep an eye on your feelings. Calmer, then? Feeling happier? Congratulations — you've just completed a meditation on the influence of the present moment. That is so simple.

Nurture Nature Yourself. Life is not like a popular dietary supplement, with people hiking happily every day. And almost anytime you go outside, you can quickly practice meditation. As you adapt to the primary rhythms of nature, your breath and thoughts slow down to match the gentle march of Mother Nature.

Only making yourself like your ten-year-old self and observing the clouds overhead will transmute stress. Extra credit if you consider heart types blowing down the shadows.

Wait not, meditate! You meet a friend, and she is delayed — again. Seek a smartphone meditation instead of wasting time tweeting and texting. Indeed, there's an application for that! Plug your ear buds, and you are all of a sudden, engaged in a 10-minute session that is oh-so-soothing. By the time you're done, bet you your friend arrives — and that you welcome her with a warm embrace instead of the "late-again" eye-roll.

Time to Fly. If you're caught in traffic, now isn't necessarily the time to "be one with your fellow riders" and surrender blissfully. You need a serene diversion. Try a mantra meditation set to create super chill music (I am a major DJ Drez fan) or invent your own ("I am love, I am light") and get lost as you walk down the lane.

Eat your favorite food Drop-Dead. Step into the kitchen with your oh-so-spiritual self and scoop up a small helping of ice cream or anything tickles your buds. This ancient tradition of mindful eating is both an essential rite of contemplation and a fantastic way of expressing appreciation for our abundance.

Meditation, meditation, and yoga and more. Truth: It is the physical poses that allow us to get into that dark, still space in our minds.

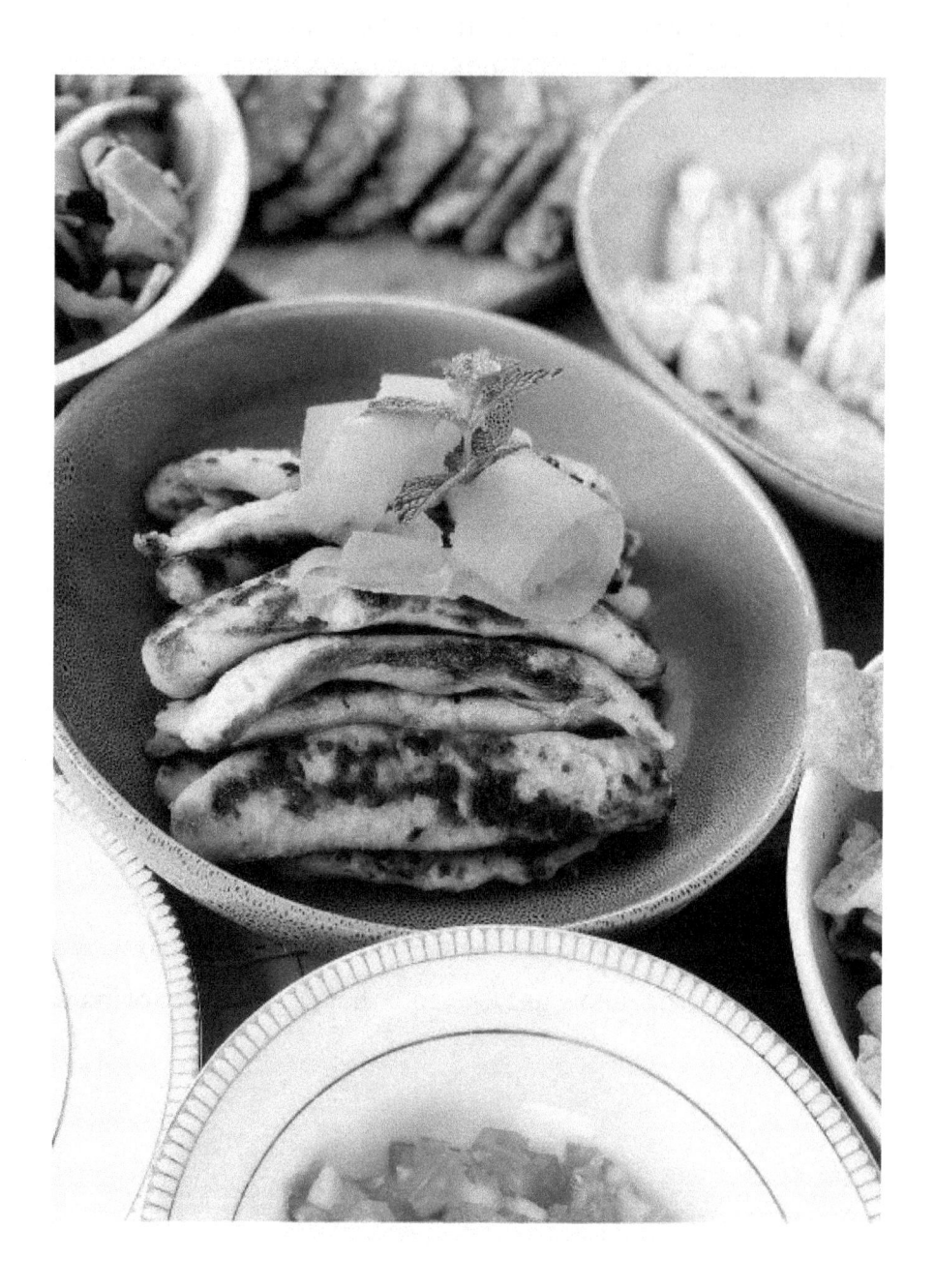

Simply Healthy Eating Habits

Have you ever asked yourself, when was the last time you went to the market to buy fruits? You go to the market most of the time, intending to buy other foods, but you hardly think of buying fruits. The fruit is very healthy, and they contain lots of nutritional benefits, especially if you are the type of person that loves sweet things. Instead of buying unhealthy things that contain a lot of sugars and calories, you can decide to buy fruits. Fruits add value to your body, and they prevent you from diseases. They contain minerals that your body needs. Now since you know that fruits are beneficial for you, the problem is that most times you tend to forget that you can eat fruits.

So, when you are hungry, you tend to munch on your favorite carbs without even searching for some fruits to eat. So, meditation will help you to be able to differentiate between right and wrong. It will help you to know that eating fruit is beneficial for your body so that you continue to eat fruits.

Foods and Drinks

Avoiding processed foods

Today there are so many processed foods in the market. The food industry is one of the fastest-growing industries today, and as the industry expands, more and more businesspeople are now trying to make money from selling processed foods. New food companies are gaining momentum and are trying to sell fast foods to people. One of the aims of these companies is to stop you from buying fruits that will not be beneficial to you. They are experts at targeting the market. They know that most of the customers in this market have low purchasing power and so they make the food cheap and enticing so that you keep on buying them.

Most of these processed foods contain many chemicals that are harmful to the body, and if you keep eating them, you will only be harming your body. If you want to achieve your ideal weight and live a healthy life, then you need to start avoiding these foods. One of the things that you need to be able to avoid processed foods is discipline. And discipline will help you to be able to make the right decisions on what you should consume and what you should not consume.

Avoiding carbs
Your meal requires just a small portion of carbohydrates, but most times, you tend to consume carbohydrates as your main meal, which then makes you gain weight. One of the major purposes of consuming carbohydrates is to give you energy.

However, when you eat them in excess, not all of them will be used as energy. Some of them will be stored as fat, and they will only make you add weight and they tend to cause sicknesses such as cardiovascular disease. So, if you want to avoid weight gain and such diseases, then it's better that you avoid eating large quantities of carbohydrates. Only eat a small portion of carbs. And make sure that you take the recommended portions of food like bread contains addictive substances, and when you eat them, they make you want to continue to eat more of them. And because of that, you will tend to eat much more than your body needs.

Eat only the recommended portion of food

Eating only the recommended portion of food means only eating the quantity of food that is meant for your body, and chronic eating disorder prevents you from doing so. When you have a chronic eating disorder, you tend to consume more food than the required portion, and many factors cause you to do so. When you are under an eating disorder, you have this belief that, if you eat a lot, you will add weight. And because of that, you keep on eating, and eating does not change your body.

Now the same thing can be applied to when you eat less than the required amount of food. It causes a huge amount of harm to your body. Skipping a meal is not good for you as well as eating too much. They are both dangerous to the body. So, the best thing that you can do is to eat the recommended amount of food that is worth it so that you will stay healthy and fit. So, with the aid of meditation, you will be able to focus and eat the correct portion of food that you are supposed to eat.

Consume plant vegetables and green food

Now, these foods contain nutrients that are very vital to the body. Most of these plant-based foods contain minerals to help your body function normally and to be able to conduct all the normal body processes. The nutrients in these foods are effective in ensuring that you maintain good health.

It also helps to provide minerals that prevent certain diseases. Some of these minerals help in boosting the metabolic processes that occur in your body. If you have not been consuming plant-based food before, then it is better to start now. Plant-based foods are very important when you're trying to lose weight; they will ensure that you only eat the right portion. If you really want to lose weight, then you should turn to plant-based food. They are very beneficial in the weight loss journey.

Our ancestors ate plant-based foods for a long time, they lived healthily, and we're happy. The paleo diet was eaten during the Paleolithic era. At that time, people eat what they planted or what they hunted. They ate the right type of food and lived a healthy life. So meditation will help you to know when to eat plant-based food and when to eliminate animal-based foods.

Eat lightly cooked food

Most times you tend to overcook your meal, and when you overcook your meal, it offers no benefits to the body, because all the nutrients in the food get lost because of the overcooking. Foods provide a lot of nutrients when they are eating raw or slightly cooked. It takes discipline to be able to cook your food slightly and not to overcook them. Sometimes you will find out that it is easier to cook food when it is fully cooked, especially with the taste that comes with it. In addition, it seems easier and sweet to consume food that has been properly cooked.

However, this kind of food will not help your body in any way. You should choose either to eat right or to enjoy your meal, and if you want to lose weight, then you should choose to eat right and eat healthily. Eating healthy is fun if you truly want to eat. Meditation will help you to set eating goals that will help you to know when not to overcook your food.

Reduce your sugar intake
Sugar is sweet and enticing, but they make you crave for more. They make you simply want more of them. Most times, you tend to crave to eat something sweet. Now eating something sweet isn't bad, but the problem is the danger that comes with it, especially when you consume them in excess. They can be very damaging to the body, so instead of being converted into energy, they are converted into fat, that is why they are very dangerous to the body and when that happens, it leads to further complications in the body.

It leads to diseases like diabetes and tooth problems. And also, they are very addictive, so with discipline, you will be able to avoid sugar, and you'll be able to regulate your sugar consumption.

You'll be able to know when to consume sugar and when to avoid it. Meditation will allow you to do that.

You will be able to decide to eat a certain amount of sugar in a day. It will help you to focus on regulating the sugar intake in your body. It will also help you to consume only the sugar that is necessary for the body, so that you will have good health and so that you will have a good body shape.

Avoid overeating

Overeating is one of the very bad habits that you must stop if you really want to lose weight. When you overeat, your body tends to add extra weight. Meditation will help you to be able to practice mindful eating. And mindful eating is essential if you want to maintain good health.

When you practice meditation, you can focus on the food that you are eating. You will be able to know that different foods have different tastes, and some foods will make you full faster at different rates than others. You will be able to analyze how your body feels after eating certain types of food, and you be able to know whether you are satisfied or not so that you will stop eating and not continue to eat. You'll be able to analyze each food and every food that you eat, and the analysis will help you to determine the portion that you should consume every day, depending on the food involved.

As a result, you will able to make well-informed decisions on the foods that you are consuming. You will be able to watch the quantity of food that you eat each day. Now, this might appear like a challenging task to do, but it is not impossible. With meditation, you'll be able to do it. Also, you'll be able to tune your mind into consuming the food that is necessary and ignore whatever is not necessary.

Drink water regularly

Water is essential in promoting good health. People that consume water tend to be healthier and happier than people that don't consume water at all. Also, consuming water will help to prevent you from certain diseases. You can also consume water by eating food that has a lot of water in them like watermelon. The greatest percentage of food is composed of water, so as you consume food, you are also consuming water. You can also decide to drink water with a glass cup. If you're not used to drinking water in the glass cup, then you can start with one or two glasses a day and increase it every day.

If you don't love drinking water, then look for things that will put in the situation to drink water. For instance, you might decide to gift yourself something after drinking a certain amount of water for the day. Drinking water isn't a big deal, and you can train yourself to drink water daily. Meditation will help you to maintain the focus that you need to be able to drink the level of water that you need each day. It will help you to create a plan for drinking water and to stick to that plan.

Program

Planning

Strategy

Tactics

METHOD

Fitness Strategies

There are two things that you should do to drop weight, and among those, we have currently covered rather extensively, which is to eat ideal and fill your body with good, clean water. The other point you have to do is get your body moving.

You don't have to buy a fitness center subscription to obtain a workout. There are several points you can do on an everyday basis that will certainly aid to kick start your body into shedding weight, and there are several workouts you can do on your own to lose weight.

When you begin working out, whether in the house or a gym, do not be discouraged if you do not see outcomes as soon as possible.

When you initially get started exercising, you can finish up with injuries, if you press your body too much. Your bones, joints, and tendons are not planned for the exertion you are putting on them. Do not assume that if you push yourself hard for a couple of exercises that you'll shed money; however, the body does not function this method. When it comes to exercising, constant and slow wins the race.

Check your weight when you begin exercising, but don't use it as a guide to accurately know how much weight you are shedding. Your weight varies throughout the day. You might just end up getting prevented if you scrutinize your weight every day.

The best way to understand if you're slimming down is by checking the fitness of your garments. One more means to know if you're reducing weight is if you can start repositioning where you typically twist your belt.

When you periodically inspect your weight and the fit of your clothing, you motivate yourself. Buy on your own some new running footwear or a brand-new pair of jeans. This will certainly assist in maintaining your motivation as you seek your weight-loss goals.

Take a day off from working out to give your body a chance to rest and repair work. Your body needs a day of rest in a week.

In succeeding day's forfeit 30 minutes daily for the workout as this will assist you in preserving your weight; however, you require a minimum of 4 days of 30-minute exercise to begin to lose weight, and five days a week is also much better.

Get necessary details on workout and note practices you can do from your own home. There are heaps of extensive study readily available on a workout, and you can pick what will certainly help you most to fulfill your fat burning objectives. Pick or surf the website some publications on wellness and conditioning from your local bookstore or collection to find out more and how to burn the preferred variety of calories you are trying to shed every week.

When your body informs you, it has had sufficient, relax. When you have functioned out for a significant quantity of time, you will certainly begin getting signals from your body. When you are just getting started in your exercise regimen, this is particularly vital.

If you decide to raise the length of your workouts, do so progressively. The same holds for the strength of your workouts.

Select an exercise regimen that suits your way of life. Everybody has a different career and a different way of living. There is no collection time that you need to or not workout. Decide the best time that suits you. If you like to exercise late before you go to bed, then do it, or if you want to apply early in the morning.

Don't stand about, stroll around. Then do it, if you can walk around. Since they are regularly moving, people that are pacers are doing themselves a lot of excellent. Pacing also helps you think.

Don't sit if you can stand. If you can stand conveniently, you will melt more calories doing so than if you were to rest. The tv and the sofa are an anti-weight loss. Do not lean on it if you are inclined to come to be a couch potato. Do not put a so comfortable chair in front of the tv so you will not invest so much time in front of it. The same holds for the computer if you're a computer addict.

If you work where you rest most time, stand and stretch every half hour or so. The majority of today's jobs are in front of a computer and need you to relax. Use the stairs instead of the elevator or escalator. These are terrific conveniences, yet they make us extremely careless. It may be quicker to take the stairways than to wait on a lift to open up.

Cigarette smoking does not add to your weight; however, it does bring about unpredictable consumption. Ten minutes of cardio a day is suitable for a lot of people, you can get this done through various other techniques than running. If you can't run for physical reasons, then attempt a 15 mins of quick walking to keep fit.

You can stroll anywhere if you have time. Take into consideration walking there or riding a bike if work or the grocery shop is not much away. It may take you longer, but you're obtaining your exercise in at the very same time.

Hide the push-button control from yourself. Remotes are also evil when it involves slimming down. If you did not have a remote, you might not even turn on the television, which suggests you might find a lot of more energetic points to do.

If you take public transport, get off a block before you quit and stroll the remaining distance. This is an excellent way to squeeze in a walk before and after work or on the way to another destination. Do pelvic revolutions to get your stomach fit. Indeed, you would not do these with anyone around, yet they are the right action in getting your body ready for more major tummy grinds.

It is also excellent on the back-muscle mass and maintains your loosened rather than limited.

Suck in your tummy when you walk. Stroll correctly, however, do your best to maintain that tummy put in. You will soon start to feel those muscles tightening.

It is impressive exactly how breathing is done correctly with your entire diaphragm, which can aid in tightening your abdominal muscles. Many people take a breath method shallow as it is, and oxygen is excellent for the brain.

Experiment with yoga exercise. Yoga is a beautiful way to reduce weight and reduce your stress and anxiety levels. Yoga exercise teaches you how to manage your muscle mass and obtain more control of your muscle mass groups.

Stamina training burns more fat than people give it credit history. When you work with structure muscle, they begin to shed fat to sustain muscle mass development. Do understand that when you acquire muscle mass, your range may not be an exact tool in establishing weight-loss because muscular tissue considers more than fat. Take the staircases two at once instead of individually. This creates you to have to exert on your own more and boost your heart price. Take your pet dog on a walk as It might be a good exercise for both of you.

Join a dance class. This could be ballroom dance where you find out dancing like the tango, fox, or salsa trot. These dancing are quick-paced and will obtain you moving. Even slow ballroom dance is a great deal of workout and will tone your legs. Or, you can take a cardio dancing course. The number of professional dancers does you recognize that are overweight?

Swim whenever you can. Swimming is an excellent method to obtain your cardio workout, and it's low to no influence on your joints, which is terrific for people who have weakening of bones or joint issues.

Try playing tennis or basketball. Playing games is an excellent means to get into shape. It's likewise extra fun to workout with another person in a competitive atmosphere. You will undoubtedly be more driven to press yourself, and you'll shed more calories, simply do not overdo it.

Always begin your exercise with a warm-up of 5-10 mins and end with cold of 5-10 mins. Your body needs to get to a particular heart price level before it positively responds well to the rest of the workout.

Don't lug your wireless phone or cellular phone with you. If it calls, walk for it. There are numerous comforts in life, and we always have everything we need at our fingertips, yet this is certainly negative for the midsection.

If you're loafing, extend your legs a bit by standing up on your toes, and after that, gradually go down to your heels. You can additionally flex your buttock muscular tissues too, but perhaps when nobody else is looking.

Before going to bed, undress, and stare at yourself before the mirror, remember what areas you require to enhance on and what areas are your ideal properties. Taking a self-inventory can keep you inspired in your workout ventures. Additionally, do not forget to match yourself on any brand-new muscle tone you might have or various other enhancements you've made.

Don't slouch in your chair. Attempt to sit up straight and erect whatsoever times. Slumping over is bad for your back and provides you with a loose and flabby figure. Make it a point to sit and stand with excellent pose always.

Most people want to target their bellies and do away with that area entirely. Sadly, we can't detect a reduction. One point you can do is a breathing exercise to help tighten those tummy muscles.

Take a deep breath as you can and tuck your belly at the same time as high as you can. Hold it for a couple of secs and afterward slowly weep. Don't allow it out so fast that your stomach flops out. This is not excellent. Try to breathe similar to this whenever you believe concerning it. About 50-60 times a day is ideal. This will assist you to shed a minimum of an inch within 20 days approximately.

Don't discourage yourself from eating and working out right by putting on garments that do not fit. Wearing the wrong kinds of clothes can make you show up more significantly than you are. This consists of workout wear also. If you put on garments that fit currently, you get to shop afterward on for smaller sized clothing, and you can sell your little-used bigger clothing in a consignment shop, or you can take them to Goodwill to be offered to a person that can use them.

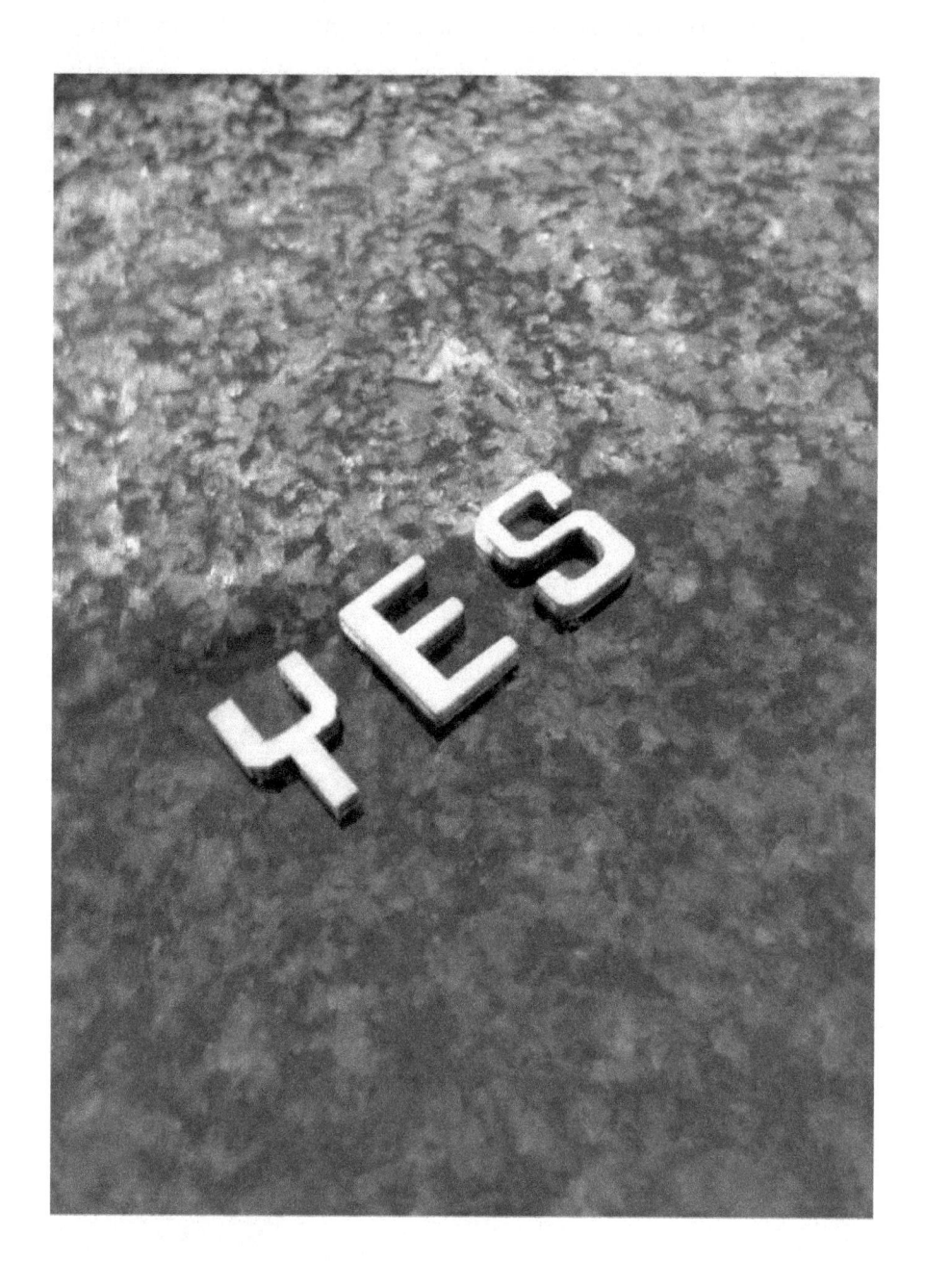

Positive Affirmations to Cut Calories

Affirmations are verbal statements that help us to affirm something we believe. So often, we say negative affirmations to ourselves without even realizing it. Recognize those negative thoughts and replace them with the positive statement that we have listed below. Repeat these to yourself daily. Write them down on a piece of paper or have notes with them on them that you leave throughout your house. Remember to practice your breathing exercises that we have learned through the other mindset exercises and keep an open mind as always.

Affirmations to Cut Calories Naturally

Cuting calories is more than just looking good to me. I understand that I need to live a healthy lifestyle to feel better all of the time.

I know how to lose weight, and I choose to do this naturally because it helps me be healthier. I know what I need to do to get the things I deserve from this life.

I am capable of reaching all of the goals that I set for myself, and I am the one who decides what I do with my life in the future.

I recognize that it's essential for me to be patient throughout this process. I can wait for the results because I know that I will get everything that I want. I do not punish myself because I don't achieve a goal as fast as I had initially hoped. I nourish myself throughout this process. I continuously look for ways to encourage myself and build my self-esteem because I know that is going to help me feel the best in the end. I can control my impulses. I know how not to act on my most significant urges. I recognize the methods that will help me to enable myself to work harder in the end. I am happy because I know how to say no.

I can turn away when confronted with an impulse. I am more durable than the biggest cravings that I have. I am proud of my ability to have a high level of willpower. I trust myself around certain foods and recognize that what tempts me does not control me.

I look at the things that I already have in my life instead of only paying attention to something that I don't have.

This is the way that will help me better achieve everything that I desire. I do not allow distractions to keep me from getting the things that I want. I can stay focused on my goals so that I can create the life that I deserve. In the end, even when I tempted by something or somebody else, I know how to push through this urge and instead focus on my goals. I will wait for everything. Love is coming to me because I know that, when it does, I will feel entirely fulfilled. I am enjoying the journey and the process that it takes to get the body that I want. I recognize that small milestones are worth celebrating.

I do not wait for one big goal to reach to be happy with myself. I look for all the methods needed to achieve greatness in this life. I understand that a temporary desire to eat something unhealthy is not worth giving up all of my goals. I know how to distract myself from my biggest cravings so that I can do something healthy instead. I recognize that doing something small is better than doing nothing at all. Even when I don't want to go to the gym, I do something at home to work out so that I can at least accomplish something minor.

Just getting started is the hardest part for me, but now I know how to work through those feelings. I am emotionally aware of what might be holding me back so that I don't allow myself to be tempted by distractions.

I control my feelings and my urges so that I don't do anything that I regret. I am happy because I am knowledgeable about the things that make me who I am.

I forgive myself when I do act on an impulse. I don't punish myself or deprive my body of the first things that it needs because I did something wrong. I sacrifice certain things that I want but never to a point where I cause punishment or torture on myself. I am successful because I am dedicated. I have strong willpower because I am successful. I move through my life with gratitude and always look to appreciate the things that I have around me. I can pick myself up when I'm feeling weak.

I am appreciative of even the hard parts of my life because they create the person that I am. I am a talented and influential person. I have control over my body, and nobody else does. I recognize my weaknesses, but in the same breath, I am very aware of my strengths. I balance my life with these things. I empower my strengths and thrive when I am in an environment that helps me grow. I recognize my weaknesses, and I always look for ways to turn them around to live happily and healthily after. I cook meals for myself because it makes me feel healthier and more reliable in the end.

I will get the dream body that I want because I can recognize things that might be healthy or unhealthy for me. I move my body at least once a day. I always feel better after I agree to a workout rather than if I try to avoid one. I can give myself rest when I need it. I don't push myself when I'm too stressed out because I know that this isn't going to help me get the things that I want.

I can always find motivation and passion within myself. I set my own goals, and I set newer and bigger ones after I achieved ones that I already completed. I do not procrastinate with my goals. I know what I have to do every day to reach these goals, and I always look for ways to go above and beyond. I am continually improving the methods that I use to live a healthy lifestyle. I self-reflect so that I can find real solutions to any issues that I might face. I don't let what other people think to take over how I see myself. I am not afraid of judgment from other people because I know that not everything negative that somebody thinks about me is right.

I make the right decision for my body. I understand that even if I make wrong decisions, sometimes, they all play a vital role in making me the person that I am today. These struggles are something that I had to undergo to become the powerful individual that I am.

I am continually losing weight because of all this dedication and passion. I feel lighter, happier, and healthier. I am free. I am pure and clean. I am collected and calm. I am peaceful, and I am so glad. I heal myself through my weight loss. I take everything wrong that I did to my body in the past and turn it into something useful, as I exercise and make healthy choices. I am always getting closer and closer to the things that I want. I'm focused on pushing through my most significant setbacks to achieve the things that I deserve. I do not sit around and fantasize about what I want anymore. Instead, I know exactly how to get this. I believe in myself because I know that this is going to be an essential part of my journey. I trust my ability actually to lose weight, and I'm not afraid of what will happen if I don't. I know how to say these affirmations to myself when I feel better.

Other people like being around me. Others recognize my hard work. Others know that I deserve to have good things in my life. When I listened to my body, I can thrive. I recognize the things that my body tells me to get the best results possible.

I feel good, and I look even better. I look great, and I look incredible because of this. Not only does losing weight help my body to look better, but it also helps my soul, and that can show through so quickly to other people. I choose to do things that are good for my body. I value myself, and I have virtue in all that I do. I add value to other people's lives, as well. I motivate myself, and therefore, I know how to motivate other people.

I am not afraid of anything. The worst thing that can happen to me is that I stop believing in myself. I will always be my best friend. I will still know how to encourage myself and include confidence in everything that I do. I love myself, and I am proud of the body that I have. I am perfect the way that I am, and I am beautiful. I am happy I am healthy, and I am free. I am focused, I center, and I am peaceful. I am stress-free and thankful. I have gratitude and love. I am attractive, and I am perfect. There is nothing that I need to punish myself. I accept everything that I am. I love myself. I am healthy. I am happy. I am free.

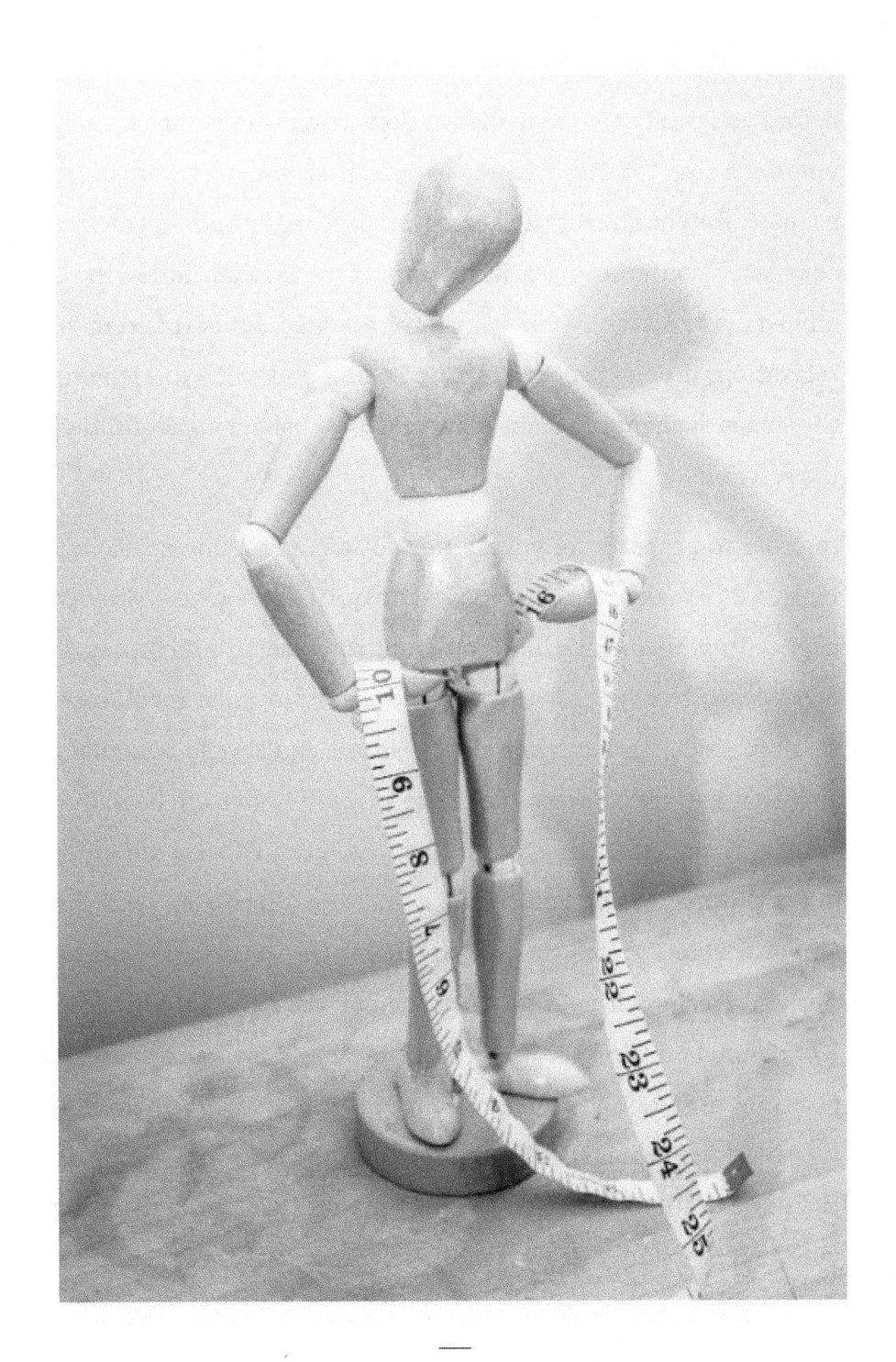

Guided Meditation for Weight Loss

Before you can begin using meditations to do things such as help you burn fat, you need to make sure that you set yourself up properly for your meditation sessions. Each meditation is going to consist of you entering a deep state of relaxation, following a guided hypnosis, and then awakening yourself out of this state of relaxation. If done properly, you will find yourself experiencing the stages of changed mindset and changed behavior that follows the session.

In order to properly set yourself up for a meditation experience, you need to make sure that you have a quiet space where you can engage in your meditation. You want to be as uninterrupted as possible so that you do not stir awake from your meditation session. Aside from having a quiet space, you should also make sure that you are comfortable in the space that you will be in. For some of the meditations, I will share, you can be lying down or doing this meditation before bed so that the information sinks in as you sleep. For others, you are going to want to be sitting upright, ideally with your legs crossed on the floor, or with your feet planted on the floor as you sit in a chair. Staying in a sitting position, especially during morning meditations, will help you stay awake and increase your motivation. Laying down during these meditations earlier in the day may result in you draining your energy and feeling completely exhausted, rather than motivated. As a result, you may actually work against what you are trying to achieve.

Each of these meditations is going to involve a visualization practice; however, if you find that visualization is generally difficult for you, you can simply listen. The key here is to make sure that you keep as open of a mind as possible so that you can stay receptive to the information coming through these guided meditations.

Aside from all of the above, listening to low music, using a pillow or a small blanket, and dressing in comfortable loose clothing will all help you have better meditations. You want to make sure that you make these experiences the best possible so that you look forward to them and regularly engage in them. As well, the more relaxed and comfortable you are, the more receptive you will be to the information being provided to you within each meditation.

A Simple Daily Weight Loss Meditation

This meditation is an excellent simple meditation for you to use on a daily basis. It is a short meditation that will not take more than about 15 minutes to complete, and it will provide you with excellent motivation to stick to your weight loss regimen every single day. You should schedule time in your morning routine to engage in this simple daily weight loss meditation every single day. You can also complete it periodically throughout the day if you find your motivation dwindling or your mindset regressing. Over time, you should find that using it just once per day is plenty.

Because you are using this meditation in the morning, make sure that you are sitting upright with a straight spine so that you are able to stay engaged and awake throughout the entire meditation. Laying down or getting too comfortable may result in you feeling more tired, rather than more awake, from your meditation. Ideally, this meditation should lead to boosted energy as well as improved fat burning abilities within your body.

The Meditation

Start by gently closing your eyes and drawing your attention to your breath. As you do, I want you to track the succeeding five breaths, gently and intentionally lengthening them to help you relax as deeply as you can. With each breath, breathe into the count of five and out to the count of seven.

Now that you are starting to feel more relaxed, I want you to draw your awareness into your body. First, become aware of your feet. Feel your feet relaxing deeply, as you visualize any stress or worry melting away from your feet. Now, become aware of your legs. Feel any stress or worry melting away from your legs as they begin to relax completely. Afterward, become aware of your glutes and pelvis, allowing any stress or worry to fade away as they completely relax simply. Now, become aware of your entire torso, allowing any stress or worry to melt away from your torso as it relaxes completely. Then, become aware of your shoulders, arms, hands, and fingers. Allow the stress and worry to melt away from your shoulders, arms, hands, and fingers as they relax completely. Now, let the stress and worry melt away from your neck, head, and face. Feel your neck, head, and face relaxing as any stress or worry melts away completely.

As you deepen into this state of relaxation, I want you to take a moment to visualize the space in front of you. Imagine that in front of you, you are standing there looking back at yourself. See every inch of your body as it is right now standing before you, casually, as you simply observe yourself. While you do, see what parts of your body you want to reduce fat in so that you can create a healthier, stronger body for yourself. Visualize the fat in these areas of your body, slowly fading away as you begin to carve out a healthier, leaner, and stronger body underneath. Notice how effortlessly this extra fat melts away as you continue to visualize yourself becoming a healthier and more vivacious version of yourself.

Now, I want you to visualize what this healthier, leaner version of yourself would be doing. Visualize yourself going through your typical daily routine, except from the perspective of your healthier self. What would you be eating? When and how would you be exercising? What would you spend your time doing? How do you feel about yourself? How different do you feel when you interact with the people around you, such as your family and your co-workers? What does life feel like when you are a healthier, leaner version of you?

Spend several minutes visualizing how different your life is now that your fat has melted away. Feel how natural it is for you to enjoy these healthier foods, and how easy it is for you to moderate your cravings and indulgences when you choose to treat yourself. Notice how easy it is for you to engage in exercise and how exercise feels enjoyable and like a wonderful hobby, rather than a chore that you have to force yourself to commit to every single day. Feel yourself genuinely enjoying life far more, all because the unhealthy fats that were weighing you down and disrupting your health have faded away. Notice how easy it was for you to get here, and how easy it is for you to continue to maintain your health and wellness as you continue to choose better and better choices for you and your body.

Feel how much you respect your body when you make these healthier choices, and how much you genuinely care about yourself. Notice how each meal and each exercise feels like an act of self-care, rather than a chore you are forcing yourself to engage in. Feel how good it feels to do something for you. For your wellbeing.

When you are ready, take that visualization of yourself and send the image out really far, watching it become nothing more than a spec in your field of awareness. Then, send it out into the ether, trusting that your subconscious mind will hold onto this vision of yourself and work daily on bringing this version of you into your current reality.

Now, awaken back into your body where you sit right now. Feel yourself feeling more motivated, more energized, and more excited about engaging in the activities that are going to improve your health and help you burn your fat. As you prepare to go about your day, hold onto that visualization and those feelings that you had of yourself, and trust that you can have this wonderful experience in your life. You can do it!

Positive Thinking Meditation

Begin in a place you feel the most comfortable and relaxed. This area should be full of positivity.

Don't use a space where you will be distracted, stressed, or bombarded with negative thoughts. For example, avoid work or common areas where you feel tension or conflict with others. It should be a personal space that means something to you and where you won't feel fear or negativity creeping in.

Close your eyes, and make sure that your body is completely relaxed.

Keep your legs straight out in front of you and arms hanging loosely by your side. If you are feeling stiff or too folded up, you won't be able to explore the positive energy coming into you.

Make sure that you are in the right mindset. You do not want to be in a mood where you are overcome or stuck on negative thinking. You have to be willing to pull yourself from these thoughts and go into a place where you can healthily and happily start feeling more positive.

Notice your breath. Don't try to transform it in any way; simply feel as the air is coming into your body and as it leaves.

Start by breathing gently and feel as your body fills with air. Allow this air to come out soft and delicately.

Don't breathe in any pattern yet. Just pay attention to how it naturally flows through you. Feel the cool air come in, and the stale, warm air come out. You are breathing in good vibes.

You are breathing in happiness, positivity, and pure energy. You are breathing out bad thoughts and feelings that are weighing you down, keeping you stuck in the same toxic mindset.

Allow yourself to heal. Allow yourself to feel positive. Remind yourself that it is okay to feel this way. Often, we don't like to stay positive because we might feel guilty. We might tell ourselves that it is not normal to feel positive when so many people in the world are angry, sad, and generally pessimistic.

That is not the way it has to be. It is perfectly acceptable for you to want to be happy. Just because other people might be living or thinking poorly does not mean that you have to allow yourself to feel this same way.

Start to count your breath now. This is how you are going to be able to focus your energy and make it easier to think positively. It's an exercise that you can apply whenever you need to change your pattern of thinking.

Breathe in. Count to five as you feel your lungs fill with air inside your body. As you breathe out, countdown from five. Let this air come out slowly. Breathe in now for one, two, three, four, and five. Breathe out now for five, four, three, two, and one. One more time, we are going to count down from ten. Breathe in for the first five and out for the last five. Continue this pattern as we finish throughout the meditation.

Ten, nine, eight, seven, six, five, four, three, two, and one.

The key to changing your mindset is by noticing the one you have now. Let thoughts naturally pass through your mind now. Notice any that might be attached to negativity.

These thoughts are natural. Let them flow in and out as easily as you would any other part of your day. Except this time, don't let the bad thoughts thrive, or even linger. Simply let it come into your mind and push it out with intention.

Pretend as though you are wading in a body of water, and the negative thoughts are like leaves or debris floating towards you. Each time a leaf gets close, push it away gently with your hand. No need to pick it up or throw it. No need to push it away forcefully. Guide this thought away lightly with your fingers.

Each time you notice one of these negative thoughts, stop yourself, and turn it around. These thoughts are fears of what might happen tomorrow. Maybe you are afraid of going into work. Perhaps you are fearful of what somebody might think or do. Maybe you are scared of a judgment call and making the wrong decision. Perhaps it is a freak accident from the past that keeps you up at night. Each time you think of something like this, gently push it away.

Negative thoughts are also regretting that linger from the past. Maybe you are always thinking about what you should or could have done differently. Perhaps you are fearful of all the things that you missed, or you can't stop thinking about one decision you made a long time ago.

Each time one of these thoughts comes into your mind, push it out with tenderness. These thoughts aren't helping you. They aren't going to make you a more productive person. They're just going to keep holding you back. It is time to move forward.

We have to focus on the 'now.' The decisions that you've made cannot be changed. Everything has already happened did so for a reason.

Notice your mindset and how you might be focusing only on the negative things. There is a dark and a light side to everything in our life. If you continuously stand in the dark, you will never be able to see all that is in the light.

Each time you have thoughts about what you do not have, remind yourself of all of the things that you do. A negative mindset is one that ignores all the chances for goodness. It is one that chooses not to see these aspects of life.

It is time to use gratitude. Gratitude is the appreciation of the things that you have in life. Both good and bad, you can find underlying gratitude. It is not about being thankful for every single thing you have. You are merely noticing how these things have a positive impact on you.

Think of something bad that has happened to you. What did you learn from this experience? What knowledge did you gain for the future? How were you able to go through this experience and still come out stronger because of it? These experiences are things that we can find benefits from, even if it was something horrible, we never wish to go through again.

There is still at least one lesson you can pull from it. Here we are just trying to find the diamond in the rough.

You are picking out that one small little beam of light through all the darkness. This does not make what happened okay, but it can help to change your mindset.

So, what lessons have you learned?

There is always something, albeit small, that is available to change your perspective for the better. It's up to you to find the gratitude in it. Continue to focus on your breathing as you notice these negative thoughts flowing away and creating a more positive mindset. Notice the negative thoughts slowing down. This makes it easier to focus on that positive energy and the bright light that beams down on your life.

Focus all of it on the good that you already have. Be ready to create more. Breathe in appreciation for everything that you have. Breathe out of any hate or anxiety you feel for the things that you don't have.

Breathe in joy and appreciation for all that surrounds us. Breathe out resentment and jealousy over people who seemingly have more than you. Breathe in the realization that you can get whatever you want. Breathe out the idea that you will be happy only when you have certain things.

Remember, we need to be incredibly appreciative of all that we have. Focus on this rather than focusing on all of the things that you still have to gain. One day, if you achieve all of these things, is that the only time that you are allowed to be happy? You should find a way to be positive, all of the time. Don't limit the moments in which you show gratitude or appreciation.

You can be a happy individual at all times in life. You do not have to wait for good things to happen to feel or show happiness. You can do this at any moment. Breathe in the idea that it is okay to be happy. Breathe out any guilt you have over having a positive mindset.

There is no endpoint for happiness.

We were taught to keep a negative outlook, believing we are destined for misery, and only show appreciation for material things or monetary gains. We were instilled with thoughts that we are only allowed to be happy at the end of hard work. Struggle, reap the benefits, repeat. But there's no time like the present to interrupt this cycle.

You do not have to live like this. You can enjoy that struggle, and you can appreciate your time as you grow in life. You do not have to wait for the end to exhale and feel whole. You do not have to wait until you have everything that you've ever wanted to be happy. You are allowed to be happy right now.

Breathe in the idea that you are going to focus more on being happy now. Breathe out the idea that we have to have things to feel good. Bad doesn't always mean, negative. Negative doesn't always mean bad. We can find appreciation from our greatest struggles. We can pull something of value out from all of the dust once it settles.

There will be struggles. A positive life is not one absent from challenge; a positive life is filled with gratitude, positivity, and appreciation for the challenge. The chance to improve.

Make a promise to yourself right now that you will do your best to power through any issue. Breathe in the idea that you're going to enjoy the journey. Breathe out the idea that you have to wait until the end of the turbulence to be happy.

Breathe in the idea that you are going to have a positive mindset throughout your entire journey. Breathe out the idea that you have to torture yourself and feel anguish over all of the challenges that you might have to endure. Focus on your breath once again. Notice as the air continues to come into your body, and how easily it leaves.

We can be grateful for this. We can have so much appreciation over the way that our bodies continue to breathe. How grateful are we that we can easily fill our bodies with air and push it out without any effort! So many individuals are not able to breathe or move as we do. This is a small thing that we can start to understand and cherish. Think about this as you breathe in again. We're going to count down from ten. Breathe in for the first five and breathe out for the last five.

Fat Burning Meditation

This fat-burning meditation is a simple 30-minute meditation that allows you to visualize your fat cells, reducing into smaller and smaller cells until they virtually vanish. Focusing on these types of hypnosis, meditations are said to help direct your subconscious mind to interact with your body so that you can begin to have a healthier and healthier body. When you focus on intentionally drawing your subconscious awareness into these activities, it encourages it to continue engaging in these activities on its own, even when you are not involved in your hypnosis session.

This is a great meditation to engage in during the day anywhere from one to three times per week, or at bedtime. They say that meditating right before you fall asleep can be particularly potent, as you are meditating during a time where your subconscious mind is particularly active. Your conscious mind is already beginning to fall asleep. During this time, you are most likely to experience the level of relaxation and receptivity needed for your subconscious mind to digest the changes you are seeking to make within it.

The Meditation

To begin this meditation, allow yourself to close your eyes and start to fade into a deep state of relaxation. Feel yourself relaxing and deeper with each breath, and notice yourself falling into a beautiful state of calmness. To help you deepen your relaxation, I will guide you through a practice that will take you to the deepest level of relaxation possible. To do this, I want you to visualize yourself standing at the top of a set of stairs. As I count down from ten to one, I want you to imagine yourself walking down that flight of stairs, taking just one step at a time. With each step, you take, visualize yourself relaxing deeper and deeper until you find yourself in a deep state of relaxation and ready to engage in a hypnotic visualization session.

Beginning with ten, visualize yourself taking a step down the stairs. Notice your surroundings, including the color of the walls, what the bottom step looks like, and any decorations surrounding you. With nine, step down again, and see yourself getting closer to the bottom of the flight of stairs. Notice your relaxation doubling with every step you take, as you step down to the eighth step. Notice how your perspective may be changing around you as you descend lower and lower down the stairs, moving down to the seventh stair. Now, step down to the sixth stair. When you are ready, step again down to the fifth stair, feeling your relaxation doubling once again as you sink deeper into a state of relaxation and calm. Now, step down to the fourth stair. As you look before you, you can see a chair coming into your view when you step down again to the third stair. As you step down to the second stair, you can see that the chair looks incredibly comfy, and you cannot wait to feel your relaxation triple when you sit in it as you step down to the first stair and then off the stairs.

When you get off the stairs at the bottom, see yourself walking up to that chair and sitting in it. Notice that this chair is the comfiest chair you have ever sat in, and upon sitting in it, you feel your entire state relaxing ten times deeper as you sink into the chair. Feel yourself becoming so calm that you can fade away in this space.

As you sit there, notice your awareness turning inward into your body. As your knowledge turns inward, draw your focus down into your fat cells. See each cell sitting there, hugging your body, and keeping you warm and comfortable in your current state. Notice how each cell feels confident that it serves a purpose, and sits proudly in its position. As you look at each of these fat cells, realize that they are not there to cause you harm or destruction, but because they genuinely believe they are meant to be there. They think they are serving an essential job for you and your life.

As you draw your awareness even closer into these cells, I want you to pick one up in your hand. See this small round cell sitting in your hand, proudly serving a purpose in your life. As you hold it, thank the cell for all that it has done, and with complete gratitude, let it know that you no longer need it to help you anymore. Cup the cell between your hands and feel it shrinking down until it vanishes between your palms.

Again, pick up another cell and hold it in your hands. With sincere gratitude in your heart, thank it for serving its purpose and let it know that you no longer need its help. Wish it well as you cup it between your palms and shrink it down until it vanishes.

Keep doing this with your fat cells as you continue to pick them up, express gratitude for their service, and then shrink them down in your palms until they vanish entirely. One by one, let each fat cell know that it is no longer needed and that you are grateful for all that it has provided you with until this point in your life. Let your remaining cells know that you now require less fat in your body to restore your health and start to feel better and better.

As you get to the end of the fat cells, notice that you look around and no fat cells remain. All you see are healthy cells that support essential functions in your body like cell regrowth, digestion, and circulation. Express sincere gratitude for every single cell in your body and its work, and allow yourself to release this perspective as you draw your awareness back into your body. See your awareness growing beyond the size of your small cells and back into the knowledge of yourself as you come back into the room where you presently sit. Feel yourself awakening from your meditation now, as you open your eyes and feel different within your body.

From now on, when you go through your daily life, notice how even though some of your fat cells continue to remain, you can almost see them disappearing. Continue to express gratitude for each cell and all that it has done to attempt to support your survival, and allow it to peacefully fade away as you allow yourself to come back into a state of lean health.

Meditation and Relaxation for Weight Loss

Anytime you walk upon a group of people meditating you know that you have come into the presence of a very positive energy, or something remarkable is happening.

Sometimes you can look and see hundreds of people sitting in silence with purpose, and nothing is happening except for extreme silence and deep thinking. It is very powerful to experience and witness hundreds of people practicing meditation at one time. It can be very motivating as well as doing something to your spirit that feels natural and great.

Even if you were to walk on a group of one hundred people and not know that they were meditating, not knowing exactly what they were doing, you would still be spiritually drawn to them, and you would feel that positive energy coming from the situation.

Your spirit would naturally be attracted to harmony and peace because it is very overpowering to see that much effort being put into sitting in silence without moving that is very powerful and intentional. Hundreds of people not moving with no agenda other than to be present in the powerful manifestation of positive energy in human goodness.

Meditating Sitting Down

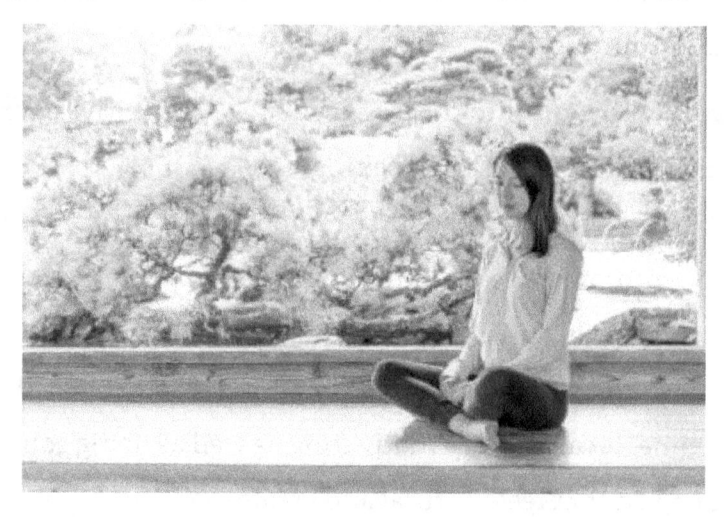

Sitting down does not just mean being seated. It means taking your seat in a relationship with the present moment, taking your stand in your life while you are sitting. Adopting and keeping a positive posture will give you pride, which will immediately change how you look and feel about yourself. Being aware of your physical sensations and thoughts while you are sitting upright is essential to meditation while you are sitting down. Whatever emotion you may have, let it flow right through you and do not let it consume you.

We can do this anytime, in any way, just make your mind aware of it and decide you want to do it. It takes many hours of practice, and you will just want to make sure that you are comfortable and totally relaxed.

Having strength and stability can come from sitting directly on the floor and crossing your legs as you do your meditating. You can also use a large pillow or cushion, which will assist in raising your butt up off the floor to a more aligned level.

This is more about being able to concentrate and focusing on keeping your mind sitting still. Just as in meditating while lying down, establish your posture, let yourself go and allow the present moment to take charge, then awareness is immediate.

Focus on the sensations of your breath in the places of the body where they are most popular to you. Your nose and your stomach are great places to focus on to practice awareness of each breath.

Focus on the feeling of each breath as it passes through your nostrils and makes your stomach rise in and out up and down. Our minds will always wander away from our primary focus to go into something it feels is more entertaining.

This will continue to happen on a regular basis because we are human, so we can just remember to acknowledge it and remind your mind to refocus on what is important at that moment in time.

Get your mind back on the thought of your breathing and begin to expand your awareness to include sensations within the body. Whatever it is that you are feeling, be aware of that, and own it. If you feel a pain in your knee, let it be known that there is a pain in that knee, the key here is to be aware of it, so that you can move on from it.

You do not have to be consumed or held as a prisoner by it. Just sit with an awareness of those sensations, acknowledge them as pleasant or unpleasant, realizing that is exactly what you are experiencing at that moment. The breath and the body come together as a complete being at this moment, and they are seen and felt as one.

You can imagine all your thoughts and emotions like the ocean flowing peacefully and calmly. Whether you are meditating or not, it can be helpful to look at this as an excuse to sit by and take in the beautiful sounds of the ocean as we stare at the wonderfully inspiring beach.

All of the time, we are present in each moment and make sure to welcome the presence of awareness to be infinite like the birds that fly in the sky. As stated before, it will take much dedication and practice to master this, but you will benefit along the way from all of your work.

Meditating While Standing

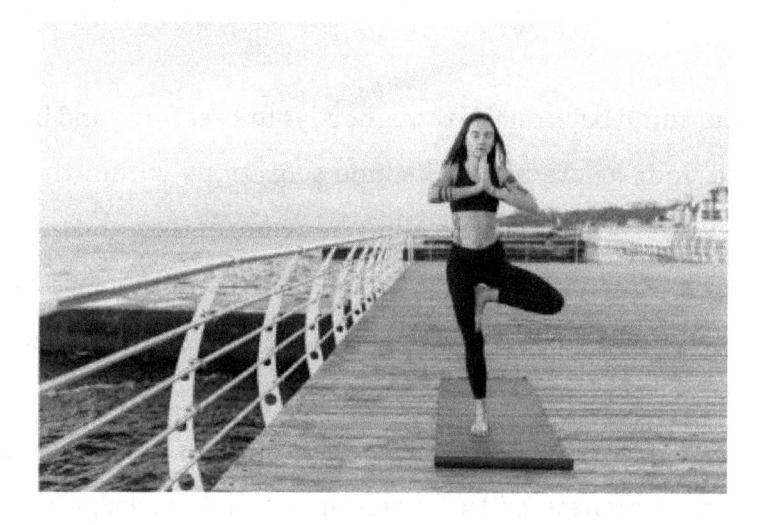

You can meditate while standing up the same way that you are able to meditate while sitting, lying down, or walking. It is one of the four popular ways in which people all over the world are now practicing their meditation.

When you think of standing meditation, it can be helpful for you to think about a tree. I know that sounds kind of silly, but the logic is that a tree has all of the knowledge and discipline that it needs to be able to stand in one place for a very long time.

Yet trees have managed to remain in a very timeless state and are still present and in the moment with us, no matter what their age seems to be. It may help your understanding of this if you go and stand beside your favorite type of tree for a while.

Try to listen and imagine hearing exactly what the tree would be hearing at that moment. You are to try to become an immediate family with the tree so that you can understand the language in which it is communicating with the universe.

You can physically experience what the tree feels by standing barefoot on the ground and becoming one with the soil. As you share the energy of tree, soil, and universe, you will begin to feel a very natural and free type of feeling in your spirit.

The same way that it is with other types of meditation, it can help if you keep up the practice for a longer period of time than you really feel like doing it. When you get that very first impulse to quit, that is when you want to focus, dig deep and keep going.

That will serve as a very vital test of your commitment, self-control, and determination. It is not easy to accomplish at first, but you will be able to do it if you just push yourself beyond each comfort zone that you try and hold onto.

Stay consistent and do not stop trying, when you can imagine yourself being completely inside of your own body, without feeling the ground touching your feet, and the sensation of your head being elevated with a sense of grace and ease looking into the direction of the Most High who is watching us all from the heavens.

Being consciously embedded in the current state of your own life and realizing that it is vital and important that you assume and retain control of your life and the direction in which it is going.

How you stand, the way that you should hold your hands, and the posture in which you need to hold your arms are all essential to this practice. Your arms should definitely be relaxed while hanging directly along each side of your body. This stance should be held for a few moments as the awareness is claimed and stood in.

You want to be sure that you align yourself and be as centered as possible because you are going to stand strong, tall, and with much dignity. Now you have the ability to surrender yourself into just simply being with what is.

Anyone can practice standing meditation anywhere, at any time, whenever they may feel like they are ready to give it a try. Some people have tried meditation, found it too difficult or boring, or just did not understand the point of it all.

We would like to welcome back those who are willing to give it another try and who are looking to make a positive change in their lives. This can be practiced literally anytime you think about doing it. It can be while you are waiting on the elevators, while you are driving, while you are waiting on the bus or train, it is all in your mind.

Meditating While Walking

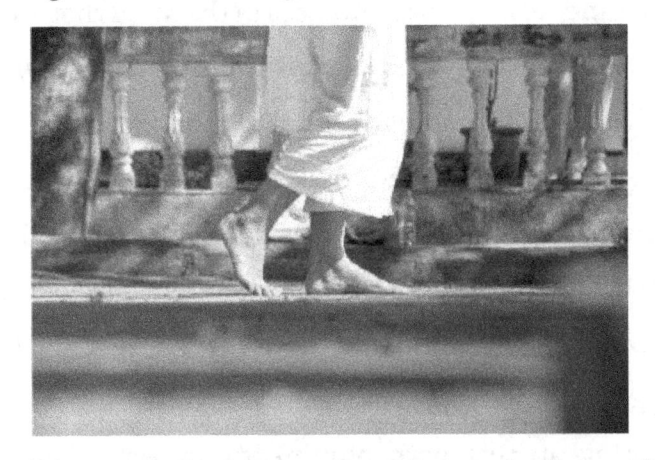

With walking, we have experienced our bodies a little bit differently than when we are sitting or lying down during meditation. Bringing our attention to our feet and using that contact between each of our feet and the ground, we can imagine it as if we are giving kisses to the world each time we step down. When the mind wanders off while we are walking and meditating, it is no different than it is with any other meditation practice. As long as we to take note of where it went and get it back into the moment, we can continue the harmony with our breathing and our steps. Take slow strides when you are walking, and you will notice more about nature and things around you.

Walking meditation can be done at many different speeds because, the same way life can throw us into another direction, our minds will assist us with the transition from mindful walking into mindful running, and that can be very a helpful tool in the practice of meditation.

You can begin by standing still, bringing awareness to your body as a whole and realize those impulses in the mind that are going to initiate the process of walking by lifting one foot, so we become aware of each time we actually lift each foot.

Now you will get the actual impulse to finally take that first step forward, which will now begin to bring us into touch with the full aspect of each sensation that we experience in our bodies that are connected with walking, lifting the heel of the foot and the actual swinging of your leg as it is being moved forward.

Coordinating all this with our breathing while being able to observe each breath as our body moves is essential to mastering this practice. While being mindful, a useful way to coordinate this is that you can breathe in as the back of your heel raises up off of the ground and breathe out each time it touches down.

Now I want you to think of what you are going to be doing with your hands during this time. You just need to be aware of the fact that they are hanging down on the side of your body and let them rest right where they are.

There is never just one specific way to accomplish these practices. You can experiment with what feels right for you and the way that you live. There is no right or wrong way; it is all about practicing, being consistent, and finding what is comfortable for you while you are walking.

Conclusion

You have learned a lot of things in this guide. You know how to release your anxiety, how to meditate properly, what the most efficient affirmations are. You can do miracles if you use these techniques properly.

The objective of this guide is to initiate you into a world of losing weight by using affirmative sentences or rather words. In this world, everyone wishes to be happy. Losing weight is just one way to reclaim your happiness back, especially if you have a more significant body. The presence of a right body image is the key to a happy life.

To achieve much in this process of weight loss, you need to embark on areas that give you a clear view of affirmations. Remember, affirmations are just phrases that are highly powerful and lead to positivity in life. By applying these affirmations, be sure that you will be able to stay focus, positive, and relaxed. There are several affirmations that you need to choose from. Try picking the ones you can manage and start your daily routine of making them permanent. Your weight will reduce tremendously.